# 30 DAYS
## to a
## Healthier
## Family

**Peggy Hughes**

SHADOW
MOUNTAIN

SALT LAKE CITY, UTAH

*This book is dedicated to my mother,*
*Mardeane Carver Jordan, and my father, Amos A. Jordan.*
*From them I must have inherited a writing bug.*

**Library of Congress Cataloging-in-Publication Data**

Hughes, Peggy J. (Peggy Jordan), 1948–
    30 days to a healthier family / Peggy J. Hughes.
      p.    cm.
    ISBN 1-57008-895-0 (Paperback)
    1. Nutrition—Popular works.   2. Children—Nutrition—Popular works.
3. Reducing diets—Popular works.   I. Title: Thirty days to a healthier family.
II. Title.

RA784.H79 2003
613.2'083—dc21    2003004430

Printed in the United States of America        72076-0024R
Publishers Printing, Salt Lake City, UT

10  9   8   7   6   5   4   3   2

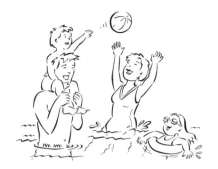

# CONTENTS

# ACKNOWLEDGMENTS

I am grateful to Wayne Westcott, Ph.D., fitness research director of the South Shore YMCA, Quincy, Massachusetts, who kindly allowed me to use his materials and advice in this book. Also, thank you to Vicky Ureuyo of the U.S. Department of Agriculture's Team Nutrition for her department's excellent resources.

I appreciate Pauline Williams, MPA, RD, CD, home economist for the Utah State University Cooperative Extension in Salt Lake City, who helped me with needed information and Rachel Johnson, RD, CD, community nutrition specialist and 5-a-Day coordinator with the Utah Department of Health's Cardiovascular Health Program, who gave me guidance and materials.

I thank my son, Evan, and my husband, John, for their cooperation and support, and my daughter, Jenny Slingerland, who modeled for the exercise photographs.

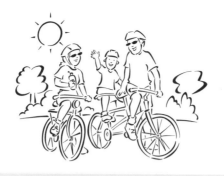

# INTRODUCTION

Health experts are warning the American public about an obesity epidemic and the news media has sounded the alarm. We are getting fatter and, of particular concern, so are our children. *People* magazine, November 4, 2002, featured a special report: "America's Overweight Kids." And the *New York Times* reported in the spring of 2002 that more than 20 percent of all preschool children are overweight, and 1 in 10 is considered obese.[1]

Doctors are beginning to see diseases in children that at one time affected primarily older adults. "Gallbladder disease among children has tripled; sleep-related breathing disruptions have quintupled; and type 2 diabetes—with its attendant risk of blindness, kidney failure, amputation, heart attack, stroke, even death—has doubled, afflicting an estimated 300,000 American youngsters."[2] High cholesterol and high blood pressure are also showing up in children as young as six years old.

Adults are in even worse shape. More than 61 percent of adults are overweight and over one-fourth of these are obese.[3] That means there are 50 million obese Americans who are prone to several life-threatening diseases, including strokes, heart disease, heart attacks, diabetes, and kidney disease.

Simply put, we are eating too much and exercising too little. There are several theories about why this is happening.

One is that we are eating away from home more often. "In 1977–78, Americans ate about 19 percent of their total calories out. By 1995, they were eating 34 percent of their calories away from home."[4] Restaurant food and prepared foods frequently have more calories, saturated fat, and cholesterol with less fiber than homemade meals. The "supersizing" trend can mean a doubling or tripling of fat and calories. When schools put in vending machines for soft drinks and high-fat snacks, the problem becomes more acute.

Another explanation for our expanding girth is the sedentary nature of today's lifestyle. Whether doing homework, driving, taking public transportation, or watching TV, we are sitting around more. Many studies correlate the number of hours watching TV to obesity.

The good news is that we are starting to realize there is a problem. In the summer of 2002, Senators Bill Frist (Republican, Tennessee) and Jeff Bingaman (Democrat, New Mexico) introduced the Improved Nutrition and Physical Activity Act to treat obesity, fund bike and walking paths, and encourage businesses to provide fitness facilities and healthier workplace food for their employees.[5] The bill did not pass but is expected to be reintroduced.

Critics of junk food are beginning to have an impact. McDonalds is the latest fast-food chain to be sued for creating obesity, and PepsiCo is exploring ways to boost the nutrition level of its snacks, including putting bits of broccoli in baked potato chips.

Solutions to the nation's health crisis can be contradictory and confusing. Some health professionals preach a high-fat, high-protein diet, while others preach a low-fat, high-carbohydrate diet. A few promote something in the middle. This book is designed to help you and your family adopt a sensible eating plan and a practical fitness plan that will energize and motivate you to a healthier life.

Discuss with family members what their objectives are in beginning a healthy eating and exercise program and how best to accomplish them. If family members are not able to do everything outlined in the 30-day plan, find out what they want to achieve and adjust the plan according to your family's circumstances. Select the ideas that work best for each person. Some may have more time and interest than others. Remember, *any healthy change your family is able to make is a positive step. Build on your successes and try to do more in the following 30 days.*

## NOTES

1. *New York Times,* March 24, 2002, WK4.
2. *People* magazine, November 4, 2002, 60.
3. *U.S. News and World Report,* August 19, 2002, 4.
4. Ibid., 43.
5. Ibid., 47.

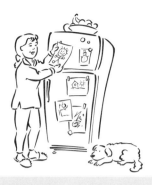

# GETTING STARTED

## A GUIDE FOR PARENTS

The 30-day plan is designed to be presented in four weekly family meetings. Each week of the program new objectives will be introduced. Each week a new food, activity, and healthy habit will be presented. Family meetings are a good time to explain basic nutrition facts, discuss fitness needs, and set or review goals. Children will benefit from a variety of fun activities that reinforce the concepts presented. A guide for these discussions and activities is provided (see pages 12–77).

Before your family begins the 30-day plan, each family member should to keep a food journal for 5 days. This is an eye-opening experience that will help your family focus on areas for improvement. A sample journal is included that you can reproduce for each person (see pages 10–11). The journal will be discussed at your first family meeting when you introduce the plan for the coming 30 days.

The healthy eating plan does not mean putting every member of your family on a weight-loss diet. Some in your family may need to lose weight to become healthier, and this book provides the necessary information to do so, but others may just need some help eating better, exercising more regularly, and making some lifestyle changes than can mean lifetime health improvements. In the back of the book is a special section for those wishing to lose weight (see page 133), as well as some advice on helping overweight children (see page 157). The simple but effective diet plan is designed to help you lose weight sensibly and keep it off and reflects sound nutritional advice. *Consult your doctor before embarking on the eating and exercise plans.*

Remember that children are not little adults. Their nutritional needs differ from the older members of your family. Children need more calcium and iron. Calcium is necessary for bone growth, and iron is needed to help them develop, prevent anemia, and help fight infections. Calcium comes from the dairy portion of the food guide pyramid. Good sources of iron are poultry, fish, lean meats, eggs, dark green vegetables, legumes, iron-fortified grain products, and iron-fortified cereals. Overall, children need adequate calories and nutrients for their growth and development.

During the first week's meeting, family members will measure their weight and fitness level. Three simple tests are given: endurance (aerobic fitness), strength, and flexibility. Younger children will enjoy doing the flexibility test, but the other tests may not be appropriate, depending on each child's age. Some family members may also want to have their blood pressure, cholesterol level, and blood sugar tested periodically.

Although 30 days is plenty of time to get a good start on becoming a healthier family, some benefits may not be immediately measurable. Therefore, you should continue the plan for another 30 days; then take the fitness tests again and continue on from there. The eating and exercise plans can be easily followed indefinitely. After all, the idea is to develop a healthier lifestyle for the long term. For those who are trying to lose weight, their scales—and their bodies—will show a difference in the first 30 days.

## TIPS FOR STAYING MOTIVATED

- ❥ Try selecting indoor and outdoor activities to add some variety.
- ❥ Grab a buddy. Exercising is always more fun with a friend.
- ❥ Join a local health club for workday workouts.
- ❥ Keep track of your mileage. Choose a vacation spot that has some nice places to walk.
- ❥ Have you met your goal? Don't forget to reward yourself.
- ❥ Bring along a Walkman to play your favorite tunes.
- ❥ Habits are much easier to keep if you enjoy them. Pick activities that you like to do.
- ❥ If you aren't too excited about a vigorous workout every day, try a more leisurely approach on some days. The important thing is to get up and get moving.
- ❥ To prevent boredom, change activity or location of activity often.
- ❥ Don't get down if you miss a chance to exercise, just do it the next time.
- ❥ Keep a record of your daily workouts.
- ❥ Get a coworker to join you for a walk.
- ❥ Buy some new exercise shoes or clothes.
- ❥ Start out slow! Over time you can increase your duration and intensity.

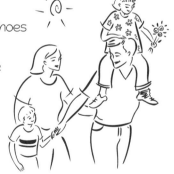

(From the Utah Department of Health Cardiovascular Program. Used by permission.)

In this book you will find healthy recipes for main meals and snacks, tips for buying and preparing food, and a calendar you can copy and use to plan meals and activities. Some of the recipes and activities are divided into the spring, summer, fall, and winter seasons. The activities are suited for children as well as teenagers. There are also ideas for expanding the eating plans and activities beyond the initial 30 days.

As you consider a healthy living plan tailored to your family's specific needs, the following ideas may be helpful:

• Ask family members to assess their eating and fitness habits and determine what they can do to improve. Encourage them to set some weekly and monthly goals, for example, "By this time next week I will have had only one soft drink." A form is provided to help them organize ideas (see page 27).

• Talk about what kinds of foods and activities your family likes, and make a list of the foods you eat most often. Look at your list and evaluate it using the questionnaire provided on page 31. Discuss how you can make those meals healthier. If anyone in your family is a vegetarian, you'll find a vegetarian food guide pyramid. If your children eat school lunch, get a copy of the month's school menus and discuss them with your family. On the basis of what you've learned, you may prefer for them to start taking lunch from home or to begin eating at the school. You may want to get involved with other parents to lobby for healthier school lunches. In June 2002, the U.S. Department of Education, the U.S. Department of Health and Human Services, and the U.S. Department of Agriculture entered into an agreement to encourage healthy eating and physical activity in school to curb obesity in children. If your children's school is not already a participating school with USDA's "Team Nutrition," talk to your principal and PTA.

• Have fun learning how to read nutrition labels. Find different foods in your home and study the labels. Some games are suggested for comparing the nutrition of various foods.

• There may be someone you know from work or someone in your neighborhood who is a doctor, a yoga instructor, a dietician, or even someone who works at a gym. Invite him or her to talk with your family and give some advice.

• Positive reinforcement can be very motivational. Blank achievement certificates are provided for you to copy (see pages 188–91). You can award weekly certificates and a special recognition at the end of each 30-day period.

• Encourage family members to post notes, quotes, pictures, and other tools to motivate each other. Reassure your family that if they slip up, they shouldn't give up. They can still make progress as long as they don't get discouraged and quit. Let other family members and friends know what you are doing so they can be supportive.

• For those family members who want to lose weight, being able to visualize their weight loss can be very motivating. Suppose one member wants to lose 20 pounds. Get a 20-pound bag of sugar and decrease the corresponding amount of sugar in the bag for every pound lost.

• Like the rest of us, teenagers are not getting enough exercise. Do whatever you can to encourage your teens to be active. Set the example. When they are about to get on the phone, recommend they meet their friend for a "walk and talk" instead. Suggest their dating activities include sports.

• If getting enough outside exercise is a challenge, consider joining a local gym or YMCA. Some gyms offer very reasonable family rates. If you want to enlist other families in your healthy living plan, you may be able to negotiate an even better rate.

• Have a TV-free day each week. In the book you'll find activities to do instead. In general, limit the amount of television everyone watches, particularly the children. You could tell your children they must "buy" TV time. Issue 30-minute coupons, no more than 2 per day, for having homework done, doing chores, choosing healthy foods, exercising, or other worthwhile criteria.

• Plan meals and make menus ahead of time.

• Eat meals as a family at least once a day. Remember that you are the one in charge of seeing to it that your family eats healthy meals. Encourage the children to take turns selecting and preparing a meal, but give them the guidelines and principles to follow when making the choice of which meals to select. Use mealtime to discuss what you all are learning and how each one feels about the program.

• A good breakfast is a must but need not be time consuming. A whole-grain cereal with fruit and low-fat milk is just fine. Breakfast provides much of a child's energy supply for the day and helps ensure that the child gets the needed daily essential vitamins and minerals. Some recipes and tips are included.

• Snacks are an important supplement to your children's meals. Because they cannot eat a lot at once, children get hungry between meals and need something to eat. Some healthy snack ideas are provided later in the book (see pages 118–25).

• Like you, children ought to be able to have candy and other sweets, but these should be eaten in small amounts and should not replace nutritious foods.

• Have snacks planned and keep lots of healthy snack foods around, especially for teenagers. Offer healthy choices: "Do you want carrots or broccoli?" Take healthy snacks on trips so you don't have to stop as often for fast food or treats.

• Don't keep soft drinks in the house. Encourage your family to drink plenty of water. Keep sports bottles of water in the fridge and refill them. You can put the family members' names on them.

• Ask your family for suggestions for fruits and vegetables each day. Check with the produce person at your super-market and find out when shipments come in. This way you can buy fruits and vegetables at their freshest, rather than after the produce has sat around for several days. If you have the space, plant a garden or try container gardening (see page 79).

• Eat out less often. When you do go to a restaurant, see how well you can do choosing healthier selections from the menu. Pick foods that are broiled instead of fried, skip the sauces, pass on the rolls and butter, and don't feel you need to clean your plate. Most restaurants serve very large por-tions, so ask for a take-out box. Request the nutrition facts if it's a fast food restaurant. Many fast food establishments now serve salads and soups. You can ask for the smallest size of fries available and share, avoid "supersizing," have a bean burrito without cheese or sauces, or have a veggie pizza. Select a sub sandwich on whole wheat with turkey and mus-tard instead of mayo and oil, or have a veggie sub. Drink water instead of soda.

• When you travel by plane, your family does not have to eat the standard fare. If you call at least one day before your flight, you can special-order healthier meals. Airlines offer low-calorie, low-cholesterol, low-fat, and low-sodium meals.

• Holidays tend to be a time to sit around and overeat. Use the time together for a physical activity, especially before the big meal. You'll tend to eat less and you'll rev up your metabolism.

• Home is the first place children learn attitudes about food and exercise. Set a good example. With almost 65 percent of adults in the U.S. over-weight, some significant lifestyle changes will need to take place in families to pre-vent children falling into the same category. Additionally, the 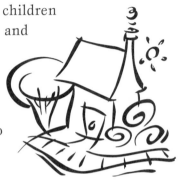 more children understand how proper nutrition and exercise help their bodies, hopefully as they get older the less likely they will be to take substances that will hurt their bodies.

• Simplify family life. One of the reasons fast food is pop-ular is that we are on the go so much that we grab whatever

## FITNESS TIPS ON BUSINESS TRIPS

➤ Take advantage of fitness facilities at your hotel.

➤ Walk instead of using the moving airport walkways.

➤ Pack hand and ankle weights for strength training on trips.

(From the Utah Department of Health Cardiovascular Program. Used by permission.)

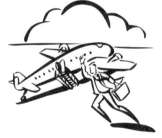

is easiest to eat. Slow down and eliminate some things that keep you in the car all the time.

• Get enough sleep and make sure your children do also. Recently doctors have stressed the importance of sleep to overall health, emphasizing that teenagers especially require more sleep than previously thought.

# FOOD JOURNAL

| | Food and Drink | Amount |
|---|---|---|
| Day 1<br>Breakfast<br>Lunch<br>Dinner<br>Snack(s) | | |
| Day 2<br>Breakfast<br>Lunch<br>Dinner<br>Snack(s) | | |
| Day 3<br>Breakfast<br>Lunch<br>Dinner<br>Snack(s) | | |
| Day 4<br>Breakfast<br>Lunch<br>Dinner<br>Snack(s) | | |
| Day 5<br>Breakfast<br>Lunch<br>Dinner<br>Snack(s) | | |

Name: _____

| Time of Day | Hunger level: not very/very | After meal: too full/ OK/still hungry |
| --- | --- | --- |
|  |  |  |
|  |  |  |
|  |  |  |
|  |  |  |
|  |  |  |

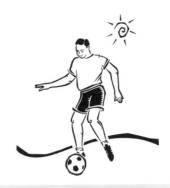

# WEEK ONE

## THE KICK-OFF MEETING

### Objectives:

- ✓ Help family members understand the food guide pyramids and the exercise pyramids.
- ✓ Introduce the concept of a healthier family in 30 days.
- ✓ Introduce the new food for the week.
- ✓ Involve everyone in a discussion of the food journals.
- ✓ Set individual goals.
- ✓ Agree on a TV-free day.
- ✓ Choose the best time of the week for meetings for discussing ideas or concerns.

### Preparation:

- ❑ Make a copy of the revised food guide pyramid, the children's pyramid (see pages 28–29), and the adult and children's exercise pyramids (see pages 34–35). Each person, especially the children, might like his or her own copy.
- ❑ Locate a set of measuring cups.
- ❑ Make a copy of the sun drawing (see page 16).
- ❑ Obtain a deck of cards.
- ❑ Make copies of the food journal questionnaire (see page 31).

❏ Be prepared to share the story of Daniel from the Old Testament (Daniel 1:5–20), if appropriate for your family.

❏ Make a copy of the chart showing calories burned by exercising (see page 36).

❏ Make copies of the personal goal form (see page 27).

❏ Complete Week One of the Four-Week Calendar (see pages 32–33) with meal plans for breakfast, lunch, dinner, and snack. Also specify a daily exercise and a weekly healthy habit and family activity.

❏ Collect seven empty boxes big enough to hold different food items. If boxes are not available, make space in your living room for seven different piles. Write the food pyramid categories on separate slips of paper.

❏ Make a copy of the fitness test form for each person (see page 37).

❏ Obtain a stopwatch or a watch with a second hand.

❏ Obtain a yardstick.

❏ Earlier in the day, slice up an apple and a pear.

❏ Get either some ascorbic acid (in the pharmacy section of a grocery store) or "Fruit Fresh."

❏ Prepare a healthy treat. Use the recipe provided (see page 25) or select one of your own.

❏ Have a TV-free activity ready to present. Use the activity idea provided (see page 26) or think up one of your own.

## Suggested Discussion:

*The Food Guide Pyramid.* Show the food guide pyramid located at the end of this chapter (see page 28). Explain that despite all the different diets that exist, the food pyramid is still a good guideline for becoming more healthy. A separate food guide pyramid for young children and another for vegetarians have been included so you can adapt the discussion to fit your family's needs. As you talk about the different categories of food in the food pyramid, compare the guidelines

## BREAKFAST IDEAS FOR "FIVE A DAY"

❧ Top cereal with fresh or dried fruit.

❧ Whirl up a fruit shake with your favorite fresh fruit, milk, and yogurt.

❧ Stir dried fruit into your muffin mix.

❧ Top your pancakes with fruit instead of syrup, or mix the fruit into the batter.

❧ Have a fresh grapefruit lightly sweetened with brown sugar or honey for breakfast or snack.

❧ Don't forget about topping yogurt with fresh or dried fruit.

❧ Top bagels or toast with pureed fresh fruit.

❧ Remember to have that glass of 100% juice for breakfast to start your day off right.

(From the Utah Department of Health Cardiovascular Program. Used by permission.)

with the information on "What Counts as a Serving" (see page 30). Your family may be surprised to learn how large or small a serving size should be.

At the base of the food pyramid are the grains. The key nutrient in grain is carbohydrates. Iron and fiber also come from grains. Have family members name as many grains as they can. The pyramid calls for six to eleven servings per day. That sounds like a lot until you consider that a serving is only half a cup, or one slice of bread, or half of a small bagel. Eleven servings may be too much for some family members. Less-active individuals, those who want to lose weight, or those who have small frames should stick to the lower number of servings. Show a ½-cup measuring cup and let someone measure that much food onto a plate to see its size. Then do the same with one cup.

*Try to make most of your servings in this category of whole grain.* For example, use 100-percent whole wheat bread instead of white bread, and use brown rice instead of white rice. Explain that the family will be introduced to different types of grains during the next few weeks.

The next row on the pyramid is divided into the fruit and vegetable groups. Start with the vegetable group and ask the family to name different types of vegetables. Tell them they will get a chance to eat some vegetables they may not have tried before. The pyramid calls for three to five servings or more of vegetables each day. A serving is ½ cup. Vegetables are so nutritious and usually so low in calories that you can encourage your family to eat as many vegetables as they like, unless they are loading the vegetables up with butter or sauces. The key nutrient in vegetables is vitamin A, but vitamin C and fiber are also found.

Fruits are packed with nutrition, although they can contain a lot of sugar and calories. The key nutrient in fruit is vitamin C, but fruit is also a good source of vitamin A and fiber. The pyramid calls for two to four servings a day. Eating more than the recommended servings of fruit is not a problem unless weight is a concern or if there are health issues that require limiting sugar intake. A serving is ½ cup or one medium-size fruit. Let everyone name as many fruits as possible and tell them they will get to try some fruits that may be new to them.

The next row on the pyramid is the milk, yogurt, and cheese group. Also on the row is the meat, poultry, fish, dry beans, eggs, and nuts group. Point out that as they move up the pyramid, the number of servings decreases, meaning they should eat fewer of these foods. One of the reasons they are to eat less of these foods is that most of them contain saturated fat. Too much saturated fat can clog up their arteries and cause heart disease. Tell them they will learn more about different kinds of fat during another week's meeting.

Two to three servings are the recommended amount to eat of the milk, yogurt, and cheese group. Children need three or four servings. The key nutrient is calcium, but other nutrients include protein, riboflavin, and vitamin D. One serving is a cup of milk, 8 ounces of yogurt, ½ cup of ice cream or frozen yogurt, and 1½ to 2 ounces of cheese. Bones need calcium in order to be strong and to grow. Ask your family if anyone can guess how many bones there are in the body. The answer is 206.

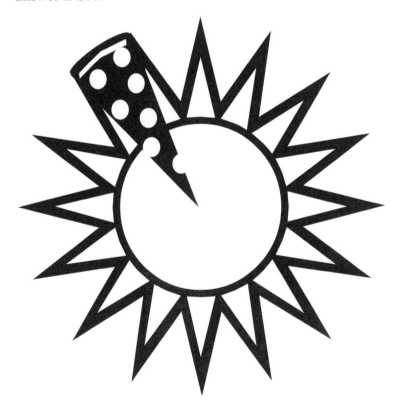

Show your family the pie-drawing of the sun and ask them if they know which vitamin is called the "sunshine vitamin." The answer is vitamin D. Explain that most of the vitamin D a body needs comes from sunlight. The rest comes from dairy foods, seafood, mushrooms, and eggs. Too little vitamin D results in weak or brittle bones, sore joints, and can also contribute to several diseases. Health experts are concerned that people are not getting enough sun, especially in the winter. Tell them they need to spend more time outdoors, but not so much that they get sunburned.

The meat, poultry, fish, dry beans, eggs, and nuts group calls for 5 to 7 ounces, not servings, daily. Three ounces of meat is considered one serving. Tell your family that a 3-ounce piece of meat is only the size of a deck of cards. If you have a deck of cards, show them how large it is and then ask them how big a piece of meat they usually eat at a meal. The key nutrient in this group is protein. Other nutrients include iron and niacin. One egg counts as a serving. Tell them they are going to try some substitutions for meat for some of their meals. A dish containing beans and a whole grain is a complete protein and can be eaten instead of meat as a way to cut down on saturated fats. The soluble fiber in beans can also lower cholesterol. Beans contain the B vitamin folic acid, potassium, and calcium.

Your family can get the benefits of meat without eating too much of it. Think of meat as a side dish and vegetables as your main dish, instead of the other way around. Prepare more casseroles, soups, stews, spaghetti sauce, salads, and stir-fry, where only small amounts of meat will be added. Eat a meatless meal a few times a week. It can be a delicious and healthy break from the everyday meat routine. Try lentil or split pea soup with cornbread or whole wheat bread; black beans and rice; chili and cornbread; corn tortillas and beans;

macaroni and cheese casserole; or baked potatoes with low-fat yogurt topping. Use nuts and seeds more often. While they are higher in fat than many other foods, the fat in nuts is the better, unsaturated type.

At the tip of the pyramid is the saturated fats, oils, and sweets group. Ask your family to name some foods that fit into this category. Suggest that they may be eating more than they should from this group. Explain that is why you would like them to have only one dessert a week. Tell them that if they participate in active sports and have eaten the recommended number of servings from the other food groups, they can have foods from the tip of the pyramid more often. Point out that some fats and oils are better for your body than others. Some oils and fats can be healthy and do not need to be eaten as sparingly. Tell them they will learn about these in a later lesson.

Recently there has been a lot of discussion among health professionals about the effectiveness of the United States Department of Agriculture's (USDA) food guide pyramid. In January 2001, the Mayo Clinic announced its own food pyramid, which is also a good one. Basically it puts unlimited amounts of fruits and vegetables at the base of the pyramid and suggests four to eight servings of grain.

*The Food Journal.* Have everyone look at their food journals and answer the questionnaire located at the end of the chapter (see page 31). Discuss the results. Tell your family their health is very important to you, which is why you think it is important that they try a plan that can make them stronger and healthier. Tell them you will try it as a family for 30 days. Get everyone's agreement on the day and time for the weekly meetings. If appropriate for your family, tell the story of Daniel in the Old Testament and point out that eating right for just 10 days made a difference in someone's

## PLAN AHEAD FOR FITNESS

➤ Set a goal for the length of time you will exercise or the distance you will cover while exercising.

➤ Don't forget to bring your walking shoes to work. Comfort is a must!

➤ Schedule a convenient time for your workday work-out and do it!

➤ Make plans to meet a coworker for a walk break.

➤ Write in your planner when you'll exercise.

➤ "Warm up" for a few minutes before getting into a fast-paced exercise.

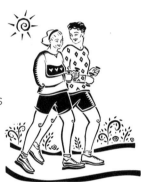

(From the Utah Department of Health Cardiovascular Program. Used by permission.)

health. Unlike the other young men in King Nebuchad-nezzar's court, Daniel and his friends refused to eat the king's rich food and drink. They were given 10 days to prove they would be healthier than the others if they ate a more simple, healthier diet. After 10 days, they in fact out-per-formed the others in physical and mental tasks (see Daniel 1:5–20).

*Exercise.* Introduce the exercise section by playing the fol-lowing game. Begin by making the statement "You know you're really out of shape when . . ."[1] As a family, try to think of creative, even silly, ways to finish the statement. Here are a few to get you started:

"You know you're really out of shape when . . ."
*You work up a sweat from pushing a pencil!*

*Your white sneakers look like new and you have been wearing them every day for a year!*

*The sack of groceries that is too heavy to lift contains bags of marshmallows!*

*Your dog takes* you *for a walk!*

*You sprain your leg muscles putting on your socks!*

Show the exercise pyramids located at the end of this chapter (see pages 34–35). Explain that children cannot always do the same exercises as adults—that is why there are two pyramids. Encourage your teenagers to develop a fitness plan for themselves using the principles you will be discussing. First look at the pyramid for adults and older children.

Everyone should start at the bottom of the pyramid and work up. Tell your family that the least amount of time should be spent in the inactive zone at the tip of the pyramid. The bottom row of the pyramid is the physical activities they do each day. Emphasize that there are ways to make daily activities more energetic. Ask for suggestions. Some ideas are walking instead of driving, taking the stairs instead of the elevator, and parking farther away from the store.

The next row of the pyramid includes sports and aerobic exercises. Have family members talk about their favorite sports or games and share how they feel after exercising. Ask if there are other sports they would like to try. Discuss sports or activities the family can do together. Always plan to wear protective gear like helmets, kneepads, and similar safety equipment, depending on the activity.

Older children and adults can do aerobic exercises. Health experts recommend at least 30 minutes a day, five days a week. If your family members are not used to exercising, they should begin gradually with 10 or 15 minutes of aerobic activity a day for a few days. Suggest that family members can pick a workout partner—a friend, parent, or sibling—

who will motivate them. Help them determine a time that fits into their schedules and encourage them to stick with that routine as much as possible. They are more likely to commit if they develop a routine. Exercises can include swimming laps, jogging or running, and brisk walking. Have family members name other aerobic activities.

At the end of the chapter is a chart showing the number of calories burned by exercising (see page 36). The word *aerobic* means "with oxygen." Tell your family that if they are exercising properly, their bodies will burn carbohydrates and fats. Oxygen will reach their muscles, where it is changed to energy. Point out that if they are breathing hard but can still carry on a conversation or sing a song while they are exercising, they are in their aerobic range.

Next on the pyramid is flexibility and strength training. Tell your family that they will learn some stretching exercises. You may also want to rent a beginner's yoga videotape. Strength training can be done with hand weights, bands, or weight machines. Free weights are often available at thrift stores, but lifters must be careful. It's best to lift in pairs so one can spot for the other. Two or three days a week is plenty. Explain that strength training will make their muscles stronger but that muscles need days off to repair themselves. Your family should start off using lighter weights or less resistance until the exercises can be done correctly and without too much effort. Then more resistance or heavier weights can be added. Some experts suggest lifting weights very slowly, for instance taking 14 seconds to perform a repetition. You can try this method and see if you get better results.

Teenage boys are often interested in weight training. Tell them that the best diet for an athlete is the type you will be discussing. Let them know they do not need to bulk up on protein to build muscles. Nor do they need protein drinks or energy drinks. Sports drinks (like Gatorade) are useful when exercising intensely for at least an hour. Sports nutritionists recommend athletes eat high-starch meals that include pasta, breads, cereals, fruits, and vegetables for energy about three hours or more before competitions.

At the tip of the exercise pyramid is the inactivity zone. Children and adults are more likely to be overweight the more time they watch TV. Tell your family they do not want to stay in this zone for very long. Ask what they can do instead.

Briefly talk to the younger children about their exercise pyramid. Please note that the strength exercises can be done by young children without using weights or bands (see page 94). There is an excellent book entitled *Strength and Power for Young Athletes,* by Avery Faigenbaum, Ed.D., and Wayne Westcott, Ph.D., which contains exercises and fitness programs for children from ages 7 to 15. Dr. Wayne Westcott has conducted studies that conclude that push-ups, pull-ups, and other exercises that are done using the body's own weight may not be as desirable as previously thought. This is because children often strain themselves doing them incorrectly. Sometimes it is better to use weights that they can easily handle with correct form.[2]

***Goals.*** Give everyone a copy of the My Goals form located at the end of the chapter (see page 27). Ask your family to think about what they would like to accomplish by the end of the 30 days. Tell them to give their answers some thought so that in the next few days they can fill out that section. Then ask them to write down a goal for the week ahead that they can reasonably accomplish. Talk about each other's goals.

*Calendar for Week One.* Show family members the calendar with the first week filled out and post it where everyone can refer to it.

## ACTIVITY: FOOD GUIDE PYRAMID

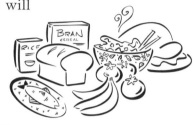

This activity for all ages will help teach your family about the food guide pyramid. Give each person a slip of paper with one of the categories from the pyramid written on it. If you have fewer children than the number of categories, just give members more than one category. Let the older children help the younger ones who can't read, or draw pictures or cut out pictures from magazines for the younger children. Place similar labels on the boxes you have collected or in a spot where you want piles to be made.

Send everyone on a "treasure hunt" to find food items in your home that fit into each food group; have them put their treasures in the right pile or box. Older children can also try a harder version. Foods like pizza, spaghetti, chili, and stew are combination foods. Have the older children categorize the combination foods. For example, spaghetti can contain foods from the meat, vegetable, and grain groups.

## ACTIVITY: FITNESS TEST

*Weight.* Those who wish should weigh themselves and record their weight.

*Flexibility.* Tape a yardstick to the floor. Have each person sit on the floor with legs straight ahead on each side of the yardstick (lower numbers should be nearest the person.) Put a piece of paper or tape at the point where your feet are extended. Write down where that point is on the ruler, because each time you take the test, you'll need to be sure your feet are at the same mark. Have the person overlap her hands, extend her arms, lower her head, and reach forward without bouncing, straining, or flexing her knees. Have her hold that position for one second while you record the farthest point reached. Take three tries and use the best score.

*Endurance (Aerobic Fitness).* You'll need a stopwatch or a watch with a second hand. Have each person (except small children) walk one mile as quickly as possible without getting winded and record the exact time in minutes and seconds.

You can measure a one-mile route in your car or go to a school track. Do this test after the 30 days and each 30-day period thereafter.

*Strength.* This test was developed by fitness expert Wayne Westcott, Ph.D. It is not necessary to use weights. You use your own body for resistance. This test is not for children or anyone with knee problems. With feet shoulder-width apart, stand 6 to 12 inches in front of a hard chair. Pretend to sit down. Cross your arms over your chest while keeping your back straight. Squat slowly until your bottom lightly touches the chair seat, then stand up slowly. Take four seconds to lower and two seconds to rise. When squatting, don't let your knees extend beyond your toes and don't bounce. Have each person do as many as possible and record the number of squats.

# TREAT:

Prepare a vegetable and fruit tray with a low-fat yogurt dip (use any low-fat yogurt as a dip for your favorite fruits and vegetables) and whole wheat crackers. Explain how the treat corresponds to the food guide pyramid.

# NEW FOOD FOR THE WEEK:

*Zucchini.* Sometime this week prepare zucchini. Use your favorite recipe or try the accompanying one.

Tell your family that zucchini contains vitamin A, vitamin C, and potassium. Vitamin A helps you see better at night, protects you from infection, and helps the cells and tissue in your body to grow and stay healthy. Vitamin C is called an antioxidant vitamin because it neutralizes the free radicals formed when the body burns oxygen, which in turn causes oxidation and cell damage in your body.

## ZUCCHINI-TUNA CANOES

2 small zucchini (each about 6 inches long)
6.5-ounce can tuna, drained, flaked
3 tablespoons salad dressing
$1/2$ teaspoon dill weed
$1/4$ teaspoon onion powder
16 (1-inch) carrot sticks

*Cut zucchini in half lengthwise. Cut a thin slice from the bottom of each half so they sit upright. Scoop out center of each half, leaving about $1/4$-inch shell; set aside. Combine tuna, salad dressing, dill weed, and onion powder. Spoon tuna mixture into zucchini halves. Cover; refrigerate and serve. Cut each "canoe" in half; insert carrot stick on each side of tuna mixture to form paddles, and serve. Makes 8 servings.*

Source: Utah State University Extension, Salt Lake County.

Show the sliced pear and apple and explain that oxidation has caused the fruit to go brown. Explain that this is kind of like what happens in your body. Now, from another apple and pear, cut some slices and dip in ascorbic acid or "Fruit Fresh." These products are essentially Vitamin C. Tell your family that this will prevent the fruits from turning brown so quickly. Vitamin C also helps heal cuts and wounds. Potassium is thought to protect against high blood pressure and helps regulate the minerals and fluids balance in your cells.

## TV-FREE ACTIVITY:

Hold a pajama party read-a-thon. As a family, pick a book to take turns reading aloud or choose someone to do the reading for the group. You can also have everyone join together in one room with their favorite book and read silently. Spend one hour or more if you'd like.

## HEALTHY HABIT:

Have dessert only once this week. For the rest of the week try a fresh fruit cup. If that is not available, canned fruit will do, provided it is packed in either water or light syrup.

### NOTES

1. *Exploring Your Body,* 4-H Cooperative Curriculum System, University of Minnesota, 46.
2. Interview with Dr. Wayne Westcott, October 22, 2002.

# MY GOALS

Name: _____

## BY THE END OF 30 DAYS MY GOALS ARE:

_____

_____

_____


## WEEK ONE GOAL(S)

_____

_____

_____


## WEEK TWO GOAL(S)

_____

_____

_____


## WEEK THREE GOAL(S)

_____

_____

_____


## WEEK FOUR GOAL(S)

_____

_____

_____

# USDA FOOD GUIDE PYRAMID

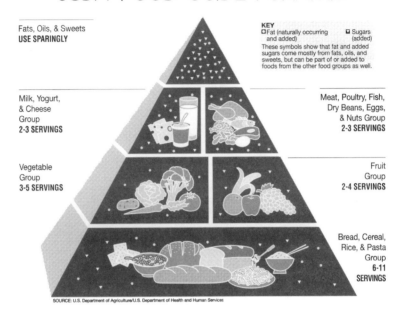

Fats, Oils, & Sweets
**USE SPARINGLY**

**KEY**
□ Fat (naturally occurring and added)    ▣ Sugars (added)
These symbols show that fat and added sugars come mostly from fats, oils, and sweets, but can be part of or added to foods from the other food groups as well.

Milk, Yogurt, & Cheese Group
**2-3 SERVINGS**

Meat, Poultry, Fish, Dry Beans, Eggs, & Nuts Group
**2-3 SERVINGS**

Vegetable Group
**3-5 SERVINGS**

Fruit Group
**2-4 SERVINGS**

Bread, Cereal, Rice, & Pasta Group
**6-11 SERVINGS**

SOURCE: U.S. Department of Agriculture/U.S. Department of Health and Human Services

# FOOD GUIDE PYRAMID FOR YOUNG CHILDREN

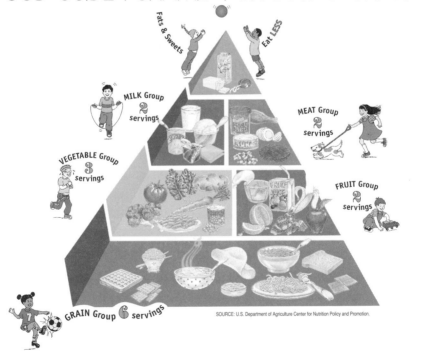

Fats & Sweets    Eat LESS

MILK Group 2 servings

MEAT Group 2 servings

VEGETABLE Group 3 servings

FRUIT Group 2 servings

GRAIN Group 6 servings

SOURCE: U.S. Department of Agriculture Center for Nutrition Policy and Promotion.

# THE VEGETARIAN FOOD PYRAMID

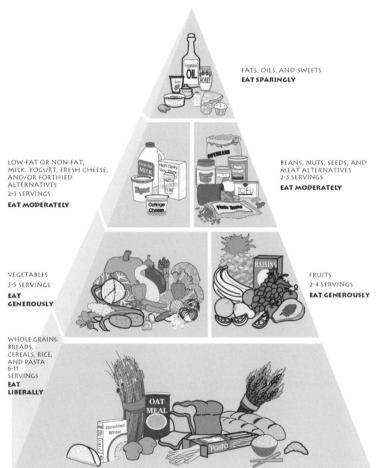

FATS, OILS, AND SWEETS
**EAT SPARINGLY**

LOW-FAT OR NON-FAT,
MILK, YOGURT, FRESH CHEESE,
AND/OR FORTIFIED
ALTERNATIVES
2-3 SERVINGS

**EAT MODERATELY**

BEANS, NUTS, SEEDS, AND
MEAT ALTERNATIVES
2-3 SERVINGS

**EAT MODERATELY**

VEGETABLES
3-5 SERVINGS
**EAT
GENEROUSLY**

FRUITS
2-4 SERVINGS
**EAT GENEROUSLY**

WHOLE GRAINS:
BREADS,
CEREALS, RICE,
AND PASTA
6-11
SERVINGS
**EAT
LIBERALLY**

General Conference Nutrition Council · 12501 Old Columbia Pike Silver Spring MD 20904 USA · tel: 301-680-6718 · fax: 301-680-6090     ILLUSTRATION BY MERLE POIRIER

# WHAT COUNTS AS A SERVING

## BREAD, CEREAL, RICE, & PASTA GROUP

1 slice of bread
½ English muffin
1 ounce ready-to-eat cereal
½ cup cooked cereal, rice, or pasta
1 tortilla
1 pancake
½ roll, bagel

## VEGETABLE GROUP

1 cup raw leafy vegetables
½ cup other vegetables—cooked or raw
¾ cup vegetable juice

## FRUIT GROUP

1 medium apple, banana, or other fruit
½ cup chopped, cooked, or canned fruit
¾ cup fruit juice
¼ cup dried fruit

## MILK, YOGURT, & CHEESE GROUP

1 cup of milk or yogurt
1½ ounces natural cheese
2 ounces processed cheese

## MEAT, POULTRY, FISH, DRY BEANS, EGGS, & NUTS GROUP

2–3 ounces cooked fish, lean meat, or poultry (use sparingly—
    3 ounces is about the size of a deck of cards)
1 cup cooked dry beans
2 eggs
4 tablespoons peanut butter
½ cup nuts

# FOOD JOURNAL QUESTIONNAIRE

Name: _____

For each day of the food journal:

Are there any food groups (except the tip of the pyramid) missing?

If yes, which ones?

Are you getting at least the minimum number of servings in each food group (except the tip of the pyramid)?

What foods could you add to your meals to help you get the recommended number of servings?

Are you eating too many servings in any food group (except vegetables)? Which foods are you eating too much of?

# FOUR-WEEK CALENDAR

| SUNDAY | MONDAY | TUESDAY | WEDNESDAY |
|---|---|---|---|
| Review for kick-off meeting. ☐ | WEEK 1 Kick-off meeting ☐<br>B.<br>L.<br>D.<br>S.<br>Exercise: | ☐<br>B.<br>L.<br>D.<br>S.<br>Exercise: | ☐<br>B.<br>L.<br>D.<br>S.<br>Exercise: |
| Review for tomorrow's meeting. ☐ | WEEK 2 ☐<br>B.<br>L.<br>D.<br>S.<br>Exercise: | ☐<br>B.<br>L.<br>D.<br>S.<br>Exercise: | ☐<br>B.<br>L.<br>D.<br>S.<br>Exercise: |
| Review for tomorrow's meeting. ☐ | WEEK 3 ☐<br>B.<br>L.<br>D.<br>S.<br>Exercise: | ☐<br>B.<br>L.<br>D.<br>S.<br>Exercise: | ☐<br>B.<br>L.<br>D.<br>S.<br>Exercise: |
| Review for tomorrow's meeting. ☐ | WEEK 4 Wrap-up meeting ☐<br>B.<br>L.<br>D.<br>S.<br>Exercise: | ☐<br>B.<br>L.<br>D.<br>S.<br>Exercise: | ☐<br>B.<br>L.<br>D.<br>S.<br>Exercise: |

B. = Breakfast     L. = Lunch     D. = Dinner     S. = Snack (optional)

| THURSDAY | FRIDAY | SATURDAY | |
|---|---|---|---|
| ☐ | ☐ | Prepare materials for next week's activities and ingredients for meals. ☐ | Healthy Habit: |
| B. | B. | B. | |
| L. | L. | L. | Family Activity: |
| D. | D. | D. | |
| S. | S. | S. | |
| Exercise: | Exercise: | Family Exercise: | |
| ☐ | ☐ | Same as above ☐ | Healthy Habit: |
| B. | B. | B. | |
| L. | L. | L. | Family Activity: |
| D. | D. | D. | |
| S. | S. | S. | |
| Exercise: | Exercise: | Family Exercise: | |
| ☐ | ☐ | Same as above ☐ | Healthy Habit: |
| B. | B. | B. | |
| L. | L. | L. | Family Activity: |
| D. | D. | D. | |
| S. | S. | S. | |
| Exercise: | Exercise: | Family Exercise: | |
| ☐ | ☐ | Plan for ongoing activities, exercise, and healthy eating ☐ | Healthy Habit: |
| B. | B. | B. | |
| L. | L. | L. | Family Activity: |
| D. | D. | D. | |
| S. | S. | S. | |
| Exercise: | Exercise: | Family Exercise: | |

Continue on for another month!

# EXERCISE PYRAMID FOR OLDER CHILDREN AND ADULTS

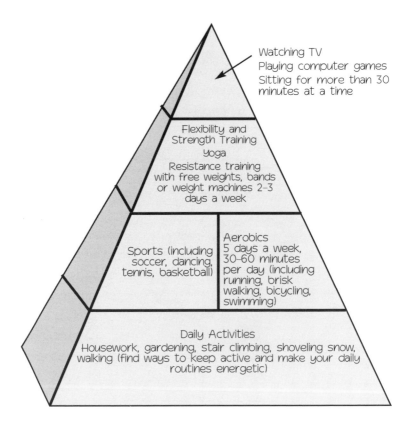

Watching TV
Playing computer games
Sitting for more than 30 minutes at a time

Flexibility and Strength Training
Yoga
Resistance training with free weights, bands or weight machines 2–3 days a week

Sports (including soccer, dancing, tennis, basketball)

Aerobics
5 days a week, 30–60 minutes per day (including running, brisk walking, bicycling, swimming)

Daily Activities
Housework, gardening, stair climbing, shoveling snow, walking (find ways to keep active and make your daily routines energetic)

# EXERCISE PYRAMID FOR CHILDREN

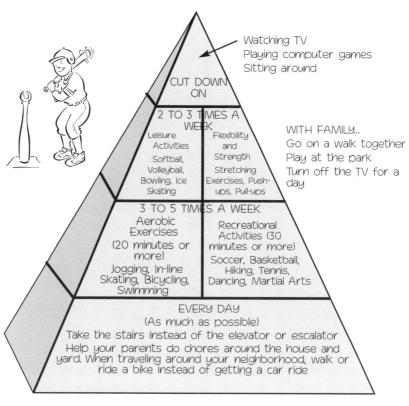

Watching TV
Playing computer games
Sitting around

**CUT DOWN ON**

**2 TO 3 TIMES A WEEK**

| Leisure Activities | Flexibility and Strength |
|---|---|
| Softball, Volleyball, Bowling, Ice Skating | Stretching Exercises, Push-ups, Pull-ups |

WITH FAMILY...
Go on a walk together
Play at the park
Turn off the TV for a day

**3 TO 5 TIMES A WEEK**

| Aerobic Exercises (20 minutes or more) Jogging, In-line Skating, Bicycling, Swimming | Recreational Activities (30 minutes or more) Soccer, Basketball, Hiking, Tennis, Dancing, Martial Arts |
|---|---|

**EVERY DAY**
(As much as possible)
Take the stairs instead of the elevator or escalator
Help your parents do chores around the house and yard. When traveling around your neighborhood, walk or ride a bike instead of getting a car ride

BY YOURSELF...
Fly a kite
Do cartwheels, somersaults, or jumping jacks
Practice sports skills

WITH FRIENDS...
Dance to music
Play games like tag and hopscotch
Join a sports team at school or at the park

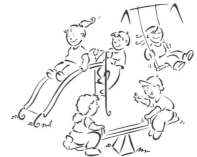

# BURNING CALORIES BY EXERCISING

| Activity | Calories burned per hour Body weight: 120 lbs. |
|---|---|
| Aerobic Dance | 330 |
| Basketball | 330 |
| Bicycling ( < 10 mph) | 220 |
| Hiking | 330 |
| Jogging | 385 |
| Racquetball | 385 |
| Running (10 mph) | 880 |
| Skating, roller | 385 |
| Skiing, cross-country | 440 |
| Skiing, downhill | 385 |
| Soccer | 385 |
| Swimming, leisure | 330 |
| Tennis | 385 |
| Walking, brisk | 220 |
| Weight training | 165 |

Source: 5-a-Day Cardiovascular Health Program, Utah Department of Health

# FITNESS TESTS

NAME_____

| WEIGHT | Day 1 | Day 30 | Day 60 | Day 90 |
|---|---|---|---|---|
| pounds: | _____ | _____ | _____ | _____ |

| FLEXIBILITY | Day 1 | Day 30 | Day 60 | Day 90 |
|---|---|---|---|---|
| stretch in inches: | _____ | _____ | _____ | _____ |

| ENDURANCE (1 mile) | Day 1 | Day 30 | Day 60 | Day 90 |
|---|---|---|---|---|
| time in min./sec.: | _____ | _____ | _____ | _____ |

| STRENGTH | Day 1 | Day 30 | Day 60 | Day 90 |
|---|---|---|---|---|
| # of squats: | _____ | _____ | _____ | _____ |

NAME_____

| WEIGHT | Day 1 | Day 30 | Day 60 | Day 90 |
|---|---|---|---|---|
| pounds: | _____ | _____ | _____ | _____ |

| FLEXIBILITY | Day 1 | Day 30 | Day 60 | Day 90 |
|---|---|---|---|---|
| stretch in inches: | _____ | _____ | _____ | _____ |

| ENDURANCE (1 mile) | Day 1 | Day 30 | Day 60 | Day 90 |
|---|---|---|---|---|
| time in min./sec.: | _____ | _____ | _____ | _____ |

| STRENGTH | Day 1 | Day 30 | Day 60 | Day 90 |
|---|---|---|---|---|
| # of squats: | _____ | _____ | _____ | _____ |

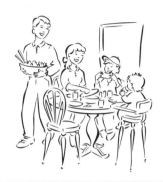

# WEEK TWO

## Objectives:

✓ Provide the family with basic information about fat and fiber, using a questionnaire to discover the amount of fat and fiber in the foods the family eats most often.

✓ Teach the family how to read nutrition labels.

✓ Determine everyone's success in meeting their goals for the first week.

✓ Discuss any problems encountered with the week's food plan and exercises.

✓ Review the school lunch menus, if applicable.

## Preparation:

❑ Select several types of foods from your kitchen to be used in the discussion and the food label activity.

❑ Make copies of the sample nutrition labels (see page 49).

❑ Make sure everyone has his goals form for the meeting.

❑ Make copies of the weekly awards for family members (see pages 188–90).

❑ Complete Week Two of the Four-Week Calendar.

❑ Make copies of the fat and fiber questionnaires (see pages 50–51).

❑ Obtain a copy of the school lunch menus.

❑ Make copies of the blank plate from the end of the chapter for everyone (see page 53) and gather some crayons or colored markers.

❑ Prepare a healthy treat (see page 47).
❑ Have a TV-free activity ready to present (see page 47).

## Suggested Discussion:

The nutrition facts label on most prepared foods will be an invaluable resource for your family as you all try to incorporate healthier food choices into your diets.

Show everyone a food item from your cupboard and point to the nutrition label. Read aloud each of the categories on the label and discuss what each means.

*Serving Size.* The serving size tells how much of the food people typically eat. The nutritional information on labels is based on the serving amount. Tell your family that if they eat more or less than the serving size shown on the label, the amount of calories, fat, and nutrients they take in goes up or down.

*Calories.* This section shows how many calories are in a single serving and how many of the calories come from fat.

*% Daily Values.* This term refers to the percentage (per serving) of the recommended daily intake of important vitamins, minerals, carbohydrates, dietary fiber, protein, fat, cholesterol, and sodium that is in a food, based on a 2,000-calorie diet. It is important to remember that some daily values are presented as minimums while others are maximums. Calcium is one example of a minimum. If a food contains only 20 percent of the daily value of calcium (based on a 2,000-calorie diet), you would need to eat *at least* five servings of that food to get enough calcium for the day. Fat, on the other hand, is a maximum. If one serving of a particular food contains 20 percent of the recommended daily value of fat, it means five servings of that food have all the fat you *should* eat in one day based on a 2,000-calorie diet. (But you should probably eat less than that if you're trying to lose weight.)

```
SMART SNACKS
```

♦ Grab fresh veggies with low-fat dip.

♦ Make air-popped popcorn or lite microwave popcorn.

♦ Add low-fat granola to fat-free or low-fat yogurt.

♦ Grab a handful of dried fruit.

♦ Keep rice cakes, pretzels, or low-fat tortilla chips and salsa on hand.

♦ Munch on cold cereal.

♦ Store graham crackers or gingersnaps at your desk.

♦ Grab a popsicle for a sweet treat.

♦ Try 100% fruit or vegetable juice to quench your thirst.

♦ Have pudding or chocolate milk made with fat-free milk.

(From the Utah Department of Health Cardiovascular Program. Used by permission.)

The daily values will change from those listed on the label if your calorie intake is higher or lower than 2,000.

***Dietary Components.*** Nutrition facts labels contain lists of nutrients that can help you judge the food's healthfulness. In most cases the goal is to get 100 percent of the daily value for the vitamins—particularly A and C—and the minerals—calcium, iron, and so on. The fat component on the label is broken down to show how much of the total fat is saturated. Stress how important it is to choose foods that are lower in saturated fat. The carbohydrates component is also divided into two important features: fiber and sugar. Look for foods higher in fiber and lower in sugar.

*Ingredients.* This section of the label lists in order by weight the ingredients in the food.

Tell everyone to pay attention to the first three ingredients listed. This will tell a lot about the food.

To help your family learn how to read and interpret food labels, have them compare the labels from two boxes of cereal. If your family primarily eats cold cereal for breakfast (using skim milk or 1 percent milk with it), tell them you would like to vary their cereals and look for ones higher in fiber and vitamins and lower in fat and sugar.

Show the labels from a box of Trix and a box of Cheerios. A copy of the labels is located on page 49. Look at the first three items in each ingredients list. Trix lists corn meal (not much fiber), and then two sugar sources, regular sugar and corn syrup. Cheerios lists whole grain oats (plenty of fiber), modified corn starch, and then wheat starch (even more fiber). Sugar is fourth on the ingredients list. Point out that Cheerios is the healthier choice of these two cereals. It has more protein, more vitamins, more fiber, and far less sugar. (A cereal with at least three grams of fiber is best.)

Tell them this does not mean they can never eat Trix or similar cereals. Trix is fortified with many vitamins and is low in fat. But as you can see from looking at the labels, plain Cheerios, which has been around for a long time, is one of the healthiest cold cereals you can feed your family. It has 110 calories, 3 grams of fiber, 1 gram of sugar, and is made from whole-grain oats, which includes the oat bran. Some "adult" cold cereals, particularly the granola kinds that are promoted as healthy, have high amounts of fat and sugar. Some granola contains 17 grams of sugar, even more than Trix.

Understanding the nutrition facts label can give your family much more control over its own health. Tell your family that making healthier food choices becomes easier when they know what nutrients their bodies need and what foods supply them. Together with the food guide pyramid and the nutrition facts label, you can teach them to plan a diet that contains the essential nutrients for good health and helps them lose weight, if necessary. Their diet needs to have adequate vitamins and minerals, which come from eating a variety of foods from the food groups.

Explain to your family that one of the most important items on the nutrition facts label. It is listed right after the calories. Ask your family members if they know what it is. The answer is fat. Each gram of fat provides 9 calories, compared to 4 calories for proteins and 4 for carbohydrates. There are 120 calories in a tablespoon of oil. In a way, that means fat is more fattening. But point out they can become overweight and unhealthy by eating too much of anything. Tell them the interesting thing about fat is that it can be very good for them or very bad. It all depends on how much fat they eat and what kind of fat they eat.

There are three basic types of fat: *monounsaturated,* which is found in olive oil, peanut oil, and canola oil; *polyunsaturated,* which is found in corn oil, safflower oil, soybean oil, and sesame seed oil; and *saturated,* which is found in meat, butter, dairy products, palm oil, coconut oil, and cocoa butter. If you have products containing some of these items, you may want to show them to your family.

Saturated fat is the least healthy of the fats. Food from animals contains mainly saturated fat. Tell your family members they can tell if a fat is saturated because it will be solid at room temperature. If you use butter, get a stick out of the refrigerator and let it sit until it is at room temperature. They will see that it is still solid. The term *omega-3 fatty acid* refers to a polyunsaturated fat found in fish, especially tuna, sardines, mackerel, and salmon, and is believed to help prevent heart disease. Explain that you would like your family to start eating more fish for this reason and to add variety to their diet. The oil found in nuts is also beneficial.

Your family should understand that besides making food taste good, fat serves a purpose in their bodies. The vitamins A, D, E, and K need fat in order to dissolve so they can get into the bloodstream. Fat also gives the body energy and provides insulation.

However, saturated fat also raises blood cholesterol levels. The body produces all the cholesterol it needs, except in the case of children under the age of two. Every time we eat food containing animal products, like meat and dairy and eggs, we

## IDEAS TO LOWER FAT INTAKE

- Use nonstick cookware and a nonfat cooking spray.
- Use skim or 1% milk.
- Read labels.
- Instead of cheddar cheese, use sharp cheddar and use half the amount.
- Use low-fat yogurt on potatoes and in dips, salad dressings, soups, casseroles, desserts, or in any recipe that calls for sour cream or mayonnaise.
- Use a non-fat butter spray or low-fat margarine for breads, potatoes, popcorn, and vegetables.
- Shop from a list to avoid buying tempting "extras."
- Stock up on recipe basics so you have ingredients on hand to cook with instead of going out.

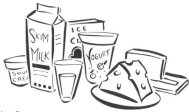

(From the Utah Department of Health Cardiovascular Program. Used by permission.)

# BREAKING DOWN CHOLESTEROL

| Form of Cholesterol | Low Risk | Moderate Risk | High Risk |
|---|---|---|---|
| Total cholesterol | Less than 200 mg/dL | 200–239 mg/dL | 240 mg/dL and over |
| LDL cholesterol | Less than 130 mg/dL | 130–159 mg/dL | 160 mg/dL and over |
| HDL cholesterol | 35 mg/dL and over | Less than 35 mg/dL | Less than 35 mg/dL |

Source: Lori A. Smolin and Mary B. Grosvenor, Nutrition: Science and Applications (2000), 143.

are taking in more cholesterol. When there is too much cholesterol in the bloodstream, fatty deposits can form in the arteries, which then slow the flow of blood through the body. This can result in a heart attack or stroke. It is a good idea for your family members to know their cholesterol levels. Higher HDL (high density lipoproteins) readings and lower LDL (low density lipoproteins) readings are desirable. The chart above indicates healthy levels of cholesterol.

HDL is sometimes called "good" cholesterol, while LDL is called "bad" cholesterol. HDL cholesterol moves quickly through the bloodstream, while LDL cholesterol moves more slowly, therefore contributing to plaque buildup in the arteries. In that sense, HDL is like a marble that speeds through the bloodstream, and LDL is like a marshmallow that sort of slogs its way through.

Point out that foods from plants (fruits, vegetables, grains) do not contain cholesterol. Also, you can easily reduce the fat content in some of your favorite recipes by using ⅓ less fat than the recipe calls for and by baking foods instead of frying. Use the chart on page 52 to compare the fat content of similar foods that are prepared differently.

*Fiber* is another term listed in the nutrition facts label. If you were a cow, your body could break down the fiber in the food you eat and convert it to energy. But human bodies cannot break down fiber small enough to be digested. Ask your family members if there is any reason to eat foods with lots of fiber. The answer is yes. Some people call fiber "nature's broom" because it can aid in digestion even though it cannot be digested itself. It moves waste along through the colon, preventing constipation and more serious problems. Fiber is found in beans, whole grains, nuts, seeds, fruits, and vegetables.

Finally, lead everyone in a discussion of how each did on his or her individual goals for the week. Gather ideas for how to improve. Hand out certificates. (Blank certificates can be found at the end of the book—see pages 188–90.)

***Calendar for Week Two.*** Show family members the calendar with the second week filled out and post it where everyone can refer to it.

## ACTIVITY: NUTRITION FACTS LABEL

Have everyone select a different packaged food from your kitchen. Take turns comparing the different features on the nutrition facts labels. For example, determine which food has the least fat, least saturated fat, most fiber, least sugar, most protein, and so on. Ask your family to discuss the healthy and less healthy components of each food and determine which of the foods are the most nutritious.

## ACTIVITY: HOW DO YOUR MEALS MEASURE UP?

Explain that studies show that people eat the same ten foods 80 percent of the time. Given that statistic, it is a good idea to look at the foods that your family eats most often. Have everyone list as many meals as they can. Then using the fat and fiber questionnaires (see pages 50–51), see how your family is doing in these two areas. You can also check on the number of fruits, vegetables, and whole grains present in the meals your family eats most often. As you analyze your family's diet and begin to think of ways to make it healthier, determine which food groups you need to eat more of and which you need to eat less of. Most families eat too few vegetables. In many homes a scoop of peas or corn at dinner is the only vegetable eaten during the day. That makes only one serving. On the other hand, when it comes to meat, families often eat the maximum number of servings or more every day.

Now get out the school lunch menus and analyze them using the same fat and fiber questions. Also compare the school lunches to the food guide pyramid. What does your family think? Should they be bringing more nutritious lunches from home some of the time?

## ACTIVITY: IMAGINING A HEALTHY MEAL

Give everyone a copy of the blank plate handout located at the end of the chapter (see page 53) and provide crayons or colored markers. Ask everyone to pretend the paper plate is an actual dinner plate; have them draw and color a healthy meal. Remind them to include the right size servings and foods from the food guide pyramid. Discuss each other's plates and the reasons each person selected those particular foods.

# TREAT:

## FRUIT YOGURT SHAKE

2 cups fresh or frozen fruit, cut up (peaches, strawberries, and
    bananas go well together)
2⅔ cups (8 scoops) nonfat frozen yogurt
4 cups cold skim milk
4 tablespoons sugar

*Put all ingredients into a blender, close the top, and puree. Pour
into chilled glasses. Makes 4 servings; adjust as necessary.*

(Source: United States Department of Agriculture, Food and Consumer Service,
Team Nutrition, Food, Family and Fun, 73; used with permission.)

# NEW FOOD FOR THE WEEK:

**Sweet potatoes.** This vegetable, going back over a thousand years, is one of the oldest in the Americas and was served at the first Thanksgiving feast. Sometime this week prepare the recipe on the next page or use one of your own. Sweet potatoes are rich in Vitamin A, an antioxidant, disease-fighting vitamin. The vegetable's yellow-orange color comes from beta-carotene, which is good at fighting cancer. Sweet potatoes also contain vitamin C, potassium, and protein.

# TV-FREE ACTIVITY:

Plan a service project in your neighborhood or community. Talk to a local community affairs person, a counselor at school, or a local charity to see how your family can help. After spending an evening planning, your family will be able to spend several TV-free days carrying out the project. Think of how much time you'll have to devote to something worthwhile if you are not watching TV.

## PINEAPPLE SWEET POTATOES

$1/2$ tablespoon margarine
2 cups fresh sweet potatoes, cooked and sliced
8-ounce can crushed pineapple in natural juice
$1/4$ teaspoon cinnamon
$1/8$ teaspoon salt

*Heat margarine in a large frying pan. Add sweet potato slices and pineapple. Sprinkle with cinnamon and salt. Simmer uncovered until most of the juice has cooked away. This may take 10 to 15 minutes. Turn potato slices a few times to coat them with the pineapple juice, then serve. Makes 4 servings.*

Source: United States Department of Agriculture.

# HEALTHY HABIT:

Skip soda pop this week. Drink water instead. If this seems too extreme, limit soda pop to once or twice a week and choose the caffeine-free, diet variety. Did you know soda pop inhibits your body's absorption of calcium? And a 12-ounce can of soda contains almost 10 teaspoons of sugar, or about 150 calories.

## TRIX®

# Nutrition Facts

Serving Size 1 cup (30g)
Servings Per Container 16

| Amount Per Serving | Trix | with 1/2 cup skim milk |
|---|---|---|
| **Calories** | 120 | 160 |
| Calories from Fat | 15 | 15 |
| | **% Daily Value **** | |
| **Total Fat** 1.5g* | 3% | 3% |
| Saturated Fat 0g | 0% | 3% |
| Polyunsaturated Fat 0g | | |
| Monounsaturated Fat 0.5g | | |
| **Cholesterol** 0mg | 0% | 1% |
| **Sodium** 200mg | 8% | 11% |
| **Total Carbohydrate** 26g | 9% | 11% |
| Dietary Fiber 1g | 4% | 4% |
| Sugars 13g | | |
| Other Carbohydrate 12g | | |
| **Protein** 1g | | |
| Vitamin A | 10% | 15% |
| Vitamin C | 10% | 10% |
| Calcium | 2% | 15% |
| Iron | 25% | 25% |
| Vitamin D | 10% | 25% |
| Thiamin | 25% | 30% |
| Riboflavin | 25% | 35% |
| Niacin | 25% | 25% |
| Vitamin B6 | 25% | 25% |
| Folic Acid | 25% | 25% |
| Vitamin B12 | 25% | 35% |
| Zinc | 25% | 30% |

*Amount in Cereal. A serving of cereal plus skim milk provides 2g fat (0.5g saturated fat), less than 5mg cholesterol, 260mg sodium, 32g total carbohydrate (19g sugars) and 5g protein.

**Percent Daily Values are based on a 2,000 calorie diet. Your daily values may be higher or lower depending on your calorie needs:

| | Calories | 2,000 | 2,500 |
|---|---|---|---|
| Total Fat | Less than | 65g | 80g |
| Sat Fat | Less than | 20g | 25g |
| Cholesterol | Less than | 300mg | 300mg |
| Sodium | Less than | 2,400mg | 2,400mg |
| Total Carbohydrate | | 300g | 375g |
| Dietary Fiber | | 25g | 30g |

**INGREDIENTS:** CORN MEAL, SUGAR, CORN SYRUP, PARTIALLY HYDROGENATED SOYBEAN AND/OR COTTONSEED OIL, MODIFIED CORN STARCH, WHEAT STARCH, SALT, GUAR GUM, GUM ARABIC, HIGH FRUCTOSE CORN SYRUP, DICALCIUM PHOSPHATE, CALCIUM CARBONATE, TRISODIUM PHOSPHATE, RED 40, YELLOW 6, BLUE 1 AND OTHER COLOR ADDED, BAKING SODA, NATURAL AND ARTIFICIAL FLAVOR, MALIC ACID, CITRIC ACID.

## CHEERIOS®

# Nutrition Facts

Serving Size 1 cup (30g)
Servings Per Container About 14

| Amount Per Serving | Cheerios | with 1/2 cup skim milk |
|---|---|---|
| **Calories** | 110 | 150 |
| Calories from Fat | 15 | 20 |
| | **% Daily Value **** | |
| **Total Fat** 2g* | 3% | 3% |
| Saturated Fat 0g | 0% | 3% |
| Polyunsaturated Fat 0.5g | | |
| Monounsaturated Fat 0.5g | | |
| **Cholesterol** 0mg | 0% | 1% |
| **Sodium** 280mg | 12% | 15% |
| **Potassium** 95mg | 3% | 9% |
| **Total Carbohydrate** 22g | 7% | 9% |
| Dietary Fiber 3g | 11% | 11% |
| Soluble Fiber 1g | | |
| Sugars 1g | | |
| Other Carbohydrate 18g | | |
| **Protein** 3g | | |
| Vitamin A | 10% | 15% |
| Vitamin C | 10% | 10% |
| Calcium | 4% | 20% |
| Iron | 45% | 45% |
| Vitamin D | 10% | 25% |
| Thiamin | 25% | 30% |
| Riboflavin | 25% | 35% |
| Niacin | 25% | 25% |
| Vitamin B6 | 25% | 25% |
| Folic Acid | 50% | 50% |
| Vitamin B12 | 25% | 35% |
| Phosphorus | 10% | 25% |
| Magnesium | 8% | 10% |
| Zinc | 25% | 30% |
| Copper | 2% | 2% |

*Amount in Cereal. A serving of cereal plus skim milk provides 2g total fat (0.5g saturated fat, 1g monounsaturated fat), less than 5mg cholesterol, 350mg sodium, 300mg potassium, 28g total carbohydrate (7g sugars) and 7g protein.

**Percent Daily Values are based on a 2,000 calorie diet. Your daily values may be higher or lower depending on your calorie needs:

| | Calories | 2,000 | 2,500 |
|---|---|---|---|
| Total Fat | Less than | 65g | 80g |
| Sat Fat | Less than | 20g | 25g |
| Cholesterol | Less than | 300mg | 300mg |
| Sodium | Less than | 2,400mg | 2,400mg |
| Potassium | | 3,500mg | 3,500mg |
| Total Carbohydrate | | 300g | 375g |
| Dietary Fiber | | 25g | 30g |

**INGREDIENTS:** WHOLE GRAIN OATS (INCLUDES THE OAT BRAN), MODIFIED CORN STARCH, WHEAT STARCH, SUGAR, SALT, OAT FIBER, TRISODIUM PHOSPHATE, CALCIUM CARBONATE, VITAMIN E (MIXED TOCOPHEROLS) ADDED TO PRESERVE FRESHNESS.

# HOW DO YOU SCORE ON FAT?

| How often do you eat | Seldom or never | 1 to 2 times a week | 3 to 5 times a week | Almost daily |
|---|:---:|:---:|:---:|:---:|
| 1. Fried, deep-fat fried, or breaded foods? | ❑ | ❑ | ❑ | ❑ |
| 2. Fatty meats, such as sausage, luncheon meats, fatty steaks, and roasts? | ❑ | ❑ | ❑ | ❑ |
| 3. Whole milk, high-fat cheeses, ice cream? | ❑ | ❑ | ❑ | ❑ |
| 4. Pies, pastries, rich cakes? | ❑ | ❑ | ❑ | ❑ |
| 5. Rich cream sauces and gravies? | ❑ | ❑ | ❑ | ❑ |
| 6. Oily salad dressings, mayonnaise? | ❑ | ❑ | ❑ | ❑ |
| 7. Butter or margarine on vegetables, dinner rolls, or toast? | ❑ | ❑ | ❑ | ❑ |

Several checks in the last two columns mean you may have a high fat intake. Perhaps you could use those types of foods less often, or in smaller quantities. Watching your fat can be a real challenge at certain meals or snacks.

Source: Food Facts for Older Adults, United States Department of Agriculture (1993), 11.

# ARE YOU GETTING ENOUGH FIBER IN YOUR DIET?

| | Seldom or never | 1 to 2 times a week | 3 to 5 times a week | Almost daily |
|---|---|---|---|---|
| **How often do you eat** | | | | |
| 1. Three or more servings of breads and cereals made with whole grains? | ❑ | ❑ | ❑ | ❑ |
| 2. Starchy vegetables such as potatoes, corn, peas, or dishes made with dry beans or peas? | ❑ | ❑ | ❑ | ❑ |
| 3. Several servings of other vegetables? | ❑ | ❑ | ❑ | ❑ |
| 4. Whole fruit with skins or seeds (berries, apples, pears, etc.)? | ❑ | ❑ | ❑ | ❑ |

The best answer is Almost daily. Whole-grain products, fruits, and vegetables provide fiber. Eating a variety of these foods daily will provide you with adequate fiber, both soluble and insoluble types.

*Source:* Food Facts for Older Adults, *United States Department of Agriculture (1993), 23.*

# MEAL COMPARISON

| HIGHER-FAT MEAL | | LOWER-FAT MEAL | |
|---|---|---|---|
| Item | teaspoons of fat | Item | teaspoons of fat |
| Fried chicken (thigh and drumstick) | 3 | Baked chicken (thigh and drumstick) | 2 |
| French fries, 10 | 2 | Baked potato, 1 med. | 0 |
| | | Margarine, 1 tsp. | 1 |
| Green beans, 1/2 c. and butter, 1 tsp. | 1 | Green beans, 1/2 c. plain | 0 |
| Whole milk, 1 c. | 2 | 2 % lowfat milk, 1 c. | 1 |
| Apple pie, 1 slice | 3 | Baked apple, 1 lrg. | 0 |
| **Total = 11** | | **Total = 4** | |

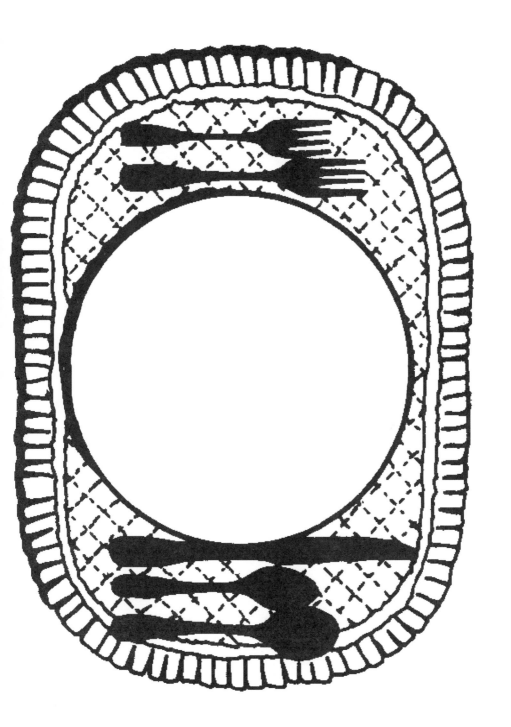

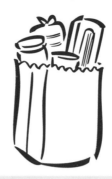

# WEEK THREE

## Objectives:

✓ To help family members understand the importance of eating "five a day."

✓ To determine everyone's success in meeting individual goals for the second week.

✓ To discuss any problems with the previous week's food plan and exercises.

## Preparation:

❏ Make sure everyone has his or her personal goals form for the meeting.

❏ Make copies of the weekly awards for family members.

❏ Complete Week Three of the Four-Week Calendar.

❏ Make a copy of the "colorful foods" chart for each family member (see page 62).

❏ Gather colored pencils, crayons, or markers.

❏ Collect small stickers.

❏ Make copies of the children's games found at the end of the chapter (see pages 63–66).

❏ Make copies of the "Fruits and Vegetables I've Tried" form (see page 67).

❏ Select small pieces of several kinds of fruits and vegetables, as many new to your family as possible.

❏ Obtain two underripe tomatoes, an apple, and a paper bag for the ripening fruit activity (see page 59).

❑ Prepare a healty treat (see page 60).
❑ Have a TV-free activity ready to present (see page 61).

## Suggested Discussion:

Explain that "five a day" means eating at least two servings of fruits and three servings of vegetables every day. Stress that this guideline provides the *minimum* amount of vitamins and minerals that help prevent diseases. Actually, family members should make an effort to eat five to nine servings of fruit and vegetables each day.

Tell them it is not as hard as it sounds, since one serving is only one-half cup of fruit or cooked vegetables, one-quarter cup of dried fruit, three-quarters cup of 100 percent juice, or one cup of salad or leafy greens. For example, you can get nearly nine servings in a day by having a glass of 100 percent fruit juice with breakfast, a banana for a snack, a salad and carrot sticks as part of lunch, cooked veggies with dinner, and a baked apple for dessert. The idea is not to eat more food, but to replace higher-calorie, high-fat foods with fruits and vegetables.

Explain how different cooking methods can either destroy or help preserve nutrients in food. Vitamins A, C, and B can be destroyed by improper cooking. Boiling vegetables leaches nutrients into the water, which is then thrown away. Foods that are exposed to high temperatures for long periods of time can also be robbed of their nutrients. Steaming and microwaving are good alternatives. Serve fruits and vegetables raw often to get the benefits of natural enzymes and phytochemicals.

Next, discuss reasons for eating more fruits and vegetables:

• Fruits and vegetables are high in fiber.
• Fruits and vegetables are low in fat.

- Fruits and vegetables are good sources of vitamins A and C and minerals like potassium, which can protect against high blood pressure.
- Some fruits and vegetables, like oranges, broccoli, peas, and spinach, are sources of folate, which protects against birth defects.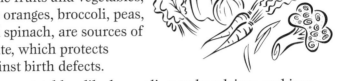
- Some vegetables, like broccoli, supply calcium and iron.
- Some vegetables, like cabbage, cauliflower, brussels sprouts, broccoli, and turnips, can protect against certain cancers.
- The soluble fiber in fruits can lower cholesterol.

Tell your family members that they may be confused when they see fruit drinks on commercials and in the grocery store. They should know that for a drink to have the amount of fruit necessary to meet the "five a day" requirements, the drink must be 100 percent real juice. They will need to read labels carefully. A drink labeled "juice drink" is often only 30 percent real fruit juice. "Fruit-flavored drink" is 10 percent or less real fruit juice; "imitation fruit drink" or "ade" is 0 percent real fruit juice, as is artificially flavored soda pop.

Explain that taking vitamin pills cannot substitute for eating fruits and vegetables; although they can be helpful if proper doses are observed. Taking a dosage that is too high, or taking too many dosages, can often have dangerous side effects. In addition, pills cannot supply the phytochemicals found in the actual fruit or vegetable. Phytochemicals (write *FIGHT-o-chemicals* on a piece of paper and show your family) are disease fighters. They are found in colorful fruits and vegetables—green, red, yellow, orange, blue, purple, and white. *Phytochemicals* means "plant chemicals." A plant produces them to protect itself from disease, and they can also protect humans who eat those plants.

## HEALTHY SNACK IDEAS

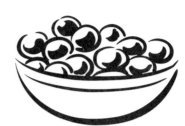

❧ Baked tortilla chips and salsa
❧ Low-sugar cereal
❧ Cheese sticks
❧ Yogurt
❧ Hard-boiled eggs
❧ Raw vegetables
❧ Cherry tomatoes
❧ Apple wedges
❧ Melon balls
❧ Mini bagels
❧ Crackers with peanut butter

(From the Utah Department of Health Cardiovascular Program. Used by permission.)

Tell family members that one way they can tell if they are getting the nutrition they need is by the color of the food on their plate. Often, the most colorful foods are also the most nutritious. The most colorful foods can also have the most antioxidant power. Antioxidants fight the damaging free radicals formed when the body burns oxygen. (Refer to pages 24–25.) Blueberries, blackberries, strawberries, oranges, cranberries, and red grapes are antioxidant leaders. So are kale, asparagus, watercress, spinach, sweet red peppers, and broccoli.

Finally, lead the family in a discussion of how each did on the individual goals for the previous week. Gather ideas for how to improve. Hand out certificates.

***Calendar for Week Three.*** Show family members the calendar with the third week filled out and post it where everyone can refer to it.

## SMART SNACKS FOR "FIVE A DAY"

❧ Keep single-serving 100% juice boxes in your car.

❧ Freeze unsweetened fruit juice into ice cubes or pops.

❧ Drink a glass of 100% fruit juice—anytime!

❧ Keep cut vegetables in cold water in the front of your refrigerator.

❧ Buy precut packages of broccoli, carrots, and cauliflower.

❧ Put fruits and vegetables out while dinner is being prepared.

❧ Put single-serving raisin boxes in your cookie jar.

❧ Use tomatoes to make a fresh salsa. Mix chopped tomatoes with minced onion, garlic, and cilantro.

❧ Prepare a berry spritzer by adding berry puree to sparkling water.

❧ Serve cut-up fruits and vegetables with a yogurt dip.

❧ Make a yummy fruit salsa using grapes, pineapples, and mangoes with brown sugar and onions.

❧ Serve cucumber slices instead of crackers with dips and spreads.

❧ Take along dried fruit as a snack.

❧ Pack an apple for your commute home.

(From the Utah Department of Health Cardiovascular Program. Used by permission.)

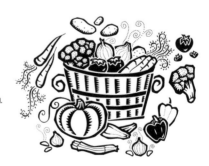

# ACTIVITY: HOW COLORFUL IS YOUR FOOD?

At the end of the chapter is a chart entitled "Colorful Foods" (see page 62). Make a copy for each member of the family. Give them crayons, colored pencils, markers, or stickers and have them mark the boxes for the fruits and vegetables they eat over the next three days.

# ACTIVITY: FRUIT AND VEGETABLE GAMES FOR YOUNGER CHILDREN

Younger children may enjoy completing the worksheets entitled "Which One Is a Vegetable?" "Which One Is a Fruit?" "Where Do They Grow?" and "Vitamins A & C," located at the end of this chapter (see pages 63–66). Have older children help the younger children complete the activity.

# ACTIVITY: FOOD TASTING

Give each family member a copy of the "Fruits and Vegetables I've Tried" worksheet found at the end of the chapter. For younger children, you may want to list or draw the fruits and vegetables they will sample in the first column. Have a sample of various fruits and vegetables on hand for your family to taste. As each food is sampled, record what it tastes like on the chart. You may want to use stickers to place in the columns.

# ACTIVITY: RIPENING FRUIT

Several fruits, including pears, peaches, mangoes, tomatoes, and bananas, are picked and often sold underripe. To demonstrate how fruit can be ripened, place an underripe tomato in a closed paper bag with a ripe apple. Leave another tomato on the counter. Over the next few days, see which tomato ripens first. Explain that the tomato in the bag ripened first because the ripe apple released a gas called ethylene, which makes fruits ripen. Bananas and apples give off this gas more than other fruits and can be used to help ripen many types of fruits. Pineapple is an exception. When you buy it, buy it ripe, because it will not ripen further.

# TREAT:

Use the following recipe or use your favorite.

## BAKED APPLES

*Heat oven to 350° F. Core enough apples for each family member, and peel a strip from the top of each apple to keep the skin from bursting.*

*Place the apples in a casserole dish. Make a mixture of raisins, brown sugar, cinnamon, and ground nutmeg to taste. You may also want to add chopped walnuts. Make enough to fill each apple. Pour ⅓ to ½ cup of unsweetened apple juice in the bottom of the casserole dish and bake for 40–45 minutes or until apples are tender. Serve warm.*

# NEW FOOD FOR THE WEEK:

**Papaya.** Papaya is a good source of vitamin A, vitamin C, and potassium. The yellow or orange skin of a papaya is not edible. The fruit inside is orange and has many black seeds. Ask the grocer to help you pick out a good one. Scoop out the seeds and cut the remaining fruit into pieces, then add bananas, berries, grapes, and pineapple chunks for a delicious fruit salad. Papayas have a tart, sweet flavor.

## TV-FREE ACTIVITY:

Check health-related Web sites found at the back of the book (see pages 185–87). Do this as a family, taking turns at the computer. If you do not have a computer at home with Internet access, take the family to the library. Make note of the Web sites that have material most useful to family members, and during the week print out the materials and discuss them together.

## HEALTHY HABIT:

Stop skipping meals, especially breakfast. Skipping meals can lower metabolism, decrease the ability to concentrate and perform well, and contribute to fatigue and overeating; it also results in missed food group servings and the nutrients they provide. Encourage family members to carry a snack with them, such as a banana or peanut butter crackers, if they think they don't have time for a meal.

# COLORFUL FOODS

## Red

Apples, beets, bell peppers, cabbage, cherries, cranberries, grapes, grapefruit, lettuce, onions, passion fruit, pears, persimmons, plantain, plums, radishes, raspberries, rhubarb, strawberries, tomatoes, watermelon

## Orange

Apricots, bell peppers, cantaloupe, carrots, clementines, kumquats, nectarines, oranges, papaya, peaches, squash, tangerines

## Yellow or White

Apples, bananas, bell peppers, cauliflower, cherries, corn, garlic, grapefruit, figs, lemons, mangoes, onions, parsnips, pears, pineapple, plums, rutabaga, squash, star fruit, sunchoke, tomatoes, turnips

## Blue or Violet

Bell peppers, blackberries, black raspberries, blueberries, cabbage, cherrries, eggplant, figs, grapes, kale, kohlrabi, plums

## Green

Artichoke, asparagus, avocado, beans, bell peppers, broccoli, brussels sprouts, cabbage, celery, chard, collard greens, cucumbers, endives, grapes, honeydew, kiwi, leeks, lettuce, limes, mustard greens, okra, onions, parsley, peas, spinach, watercress

## Totals

# WHICH ONE IS A VEGETABLE?

CIRCLE THE VEGETABLES.

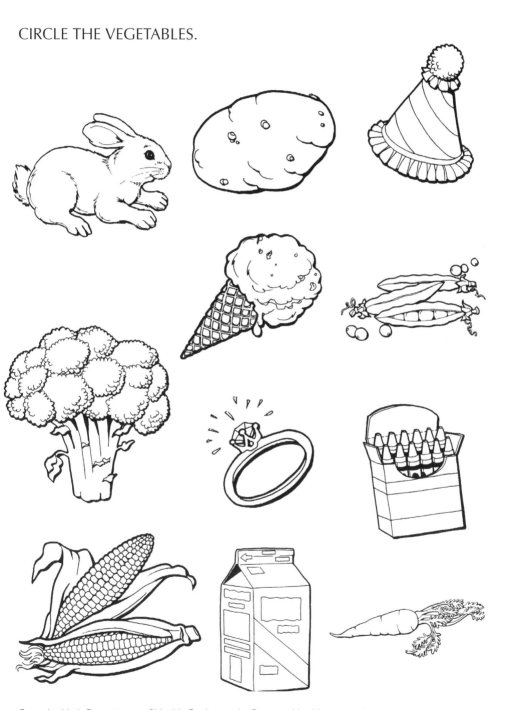

# WHICH ONE IS A FRUIT?

CIRCLE THE FRUITS.

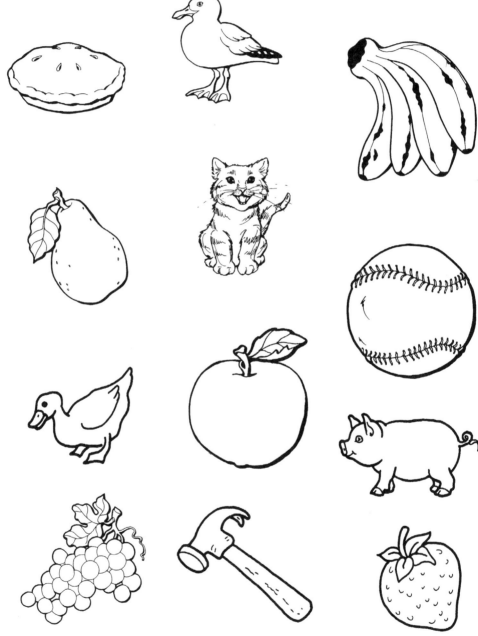

# WHERE DO THEY GROW?

DRAW A LINE FROM EACH FOOD THAT GROWS ON A VINE OR
A BUSH TO THE PICTURE OF A VINE.

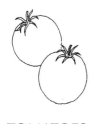

TOMATOES

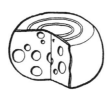

WAGON

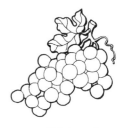

GRAPES

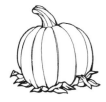

PUMPKIN

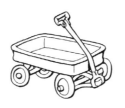

CHEESE

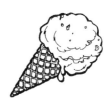

ICE CREAM

*From the Utah Department of Health Cardiovascular Program. Used by permission.*

# VITAMINS A & C

CAN YOU NAME THE FRUITS AND VEGETABLES IN THE
PICTURES? CHOOSE FROM THE LIST BELOW.

BROCCOLI   PINEAPPLE   LETTUCE
ORANGE    CARROT    STRAWBERRY
TOMATO    PEACH

THESE FRUITS AND VEGETABLES HAVE VITAMIN A. THEY HELP
OUR EYES SEE BETTER.

THESE FRUITS AND VEGETABLES HAVE VITAMIN C. THEY HELP
OUR CUTS HEAL.

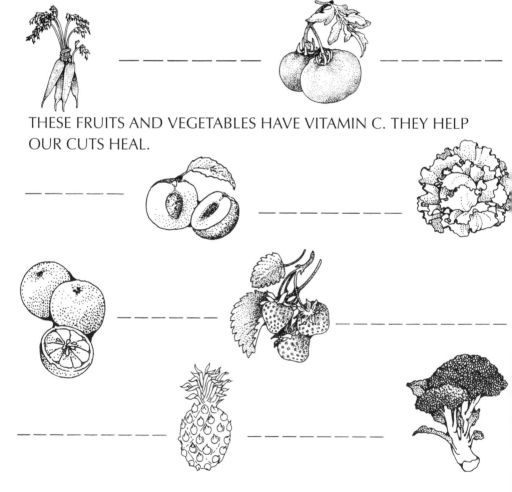

*From the Utah Department of Health Cardiovascular Program. Used by permission.*

# FRUITS AND VEGETABLES I TRIED

| Fruit or vegetable | I tried it | Tastes yummy | Tastes OK | Sweet | Sour | I don't know |
|---|---|---|---|---|---|---|
|  |  |  |  |  |  |  |
|  |  |  |  |  |  |  |
|  |  |  |  |  |  |  |
|  |  |  |  |  |  |  |
|  |  |  |  |  |  |  |
|  |  |  |  |  |  |  |
|  |  |  |  |  |  |  |

*From the Utah Department of Health Cardiovascular Program. Used by permission.*

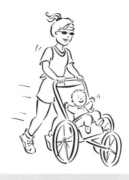

# WEEK FOUR

## THE WRAP UP

### Objectives:

✓ Retake fitness tests at the end of the week.
✓ Determine everyone's success in meeting their goals for the third week.
✓ Discuss any problems with the week's food plan and exercises.
✓ Review what makes a healthy food.
✓ Discuss calories and weight loss or gain.
✓ Briefly discuss sports nutrition.
✓ Analyze the past 30 days and discuss what worked, what didn't work, what was difficult, and what could be modified.
✓ Encourage everyone to continue healthy eating and exercise for another 30 days.
✓ Award special recognition certificates.

### Preparation:

❑ Make sure everyone has his or her personal goals form.
❑ Prepare special recognition certificates (see pages 188–91).
❑ Complete Week Four of the Four-Week Calendar.
❑ Locate a stopwatch or a watch with a second hand.
❑ Obtain a yardstick.

❑ Make sure everyone has previous fitness scores.

❑ Collect nutrition facts labels from several types of foods.

❑ Prepare balloons with slips of paper for the Balloon Pop activity (see page 74).

❑ Prepare a healthy treat (see page 75).

❑ Have storage containers ready for the TV-free activity.

❑ Obtain acid-free plastic document sleeves.

## Suggested Discussion:

Tell your family members you are going to talk a little about calories. The more calories in a food, the more energy it contains and the longer it takes for the body to burn that food off or digest it.

Maintaining weight, gaining weight, or losing weight is as simple as "calories in, calories out." If you eat the same amount of calories as you burn during the day, your weight will stay the same. If you eat more calories than your body needs to perform its activities, your body will store the calories as fat and you will gain weight. If you eat less than your body needs, you will lose weight because your body will use its stored fat for energy.

Another way for the body to use stored fat and lose weight is to increase the body's energy needs. This can be done by exercising. Give the following example:

Pretend that (name a child) eats only one ounce of potato chips. It amounts to 150 calories. If (name the child) takes a brisk walk for about 30 minutes, his or her body will use 150 calories. In other words, the energy balance is equal and (name the child)'s weight is unchanged.

One pound of fat is equal to 3,500 calories. So consuming 500 extra calories a day will result in a weight gain of about 1 pound per week or 52 pounds a year. Eating 250 extra calories a day will cause you to gain half a pound a week or 26 pounds a year. To put this in perspective, a can of soda pop is

## TIPS FOR EATING OUT

❥ Share an entrée or ask for a take-out box with your order. Put half in the box before you begin eating so you won't be tempted by large portions.

❥ Ask for substitutions such as a baked potato or fresh fruit for French fries, coleslaw, or other high-fat side dishes.

❥ Be careful at the salad bar. Limit high-fat toppings such as cheese, meats, creamy dressings, nuts, and seeds. Choose more veggies and fruit.

❥ Ask for the dressing on the side. Use the "fork method" and dip the tongs of the fork into the dressing and then into your salad.

❥ Choose foods that are naturally lower in fat (fish, poultry, or seafood), or that have been prepared with low-fat cooking methods, not fried.

❥ Select foods that aren't cooked in creamy sauces.

❥ Ask for sour cream, butter, and dressing on the side.

❥ Share a dessert rather than eating the whole serving.

❥ Don't be afraid to make requests and ask for low-fat modifications.

❥ Allow yourself to indulge in high-fat favorites on special occasions only (your birthday, a special holiday), not every time you go out.

(From the Utah Department of Health Cardiovascular Program. Used by permission.)

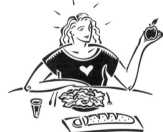

150 calories and just 14 fries is 225 calories. It's easy to see how extra calories can add up and the weight pile on, especially when the body isn't using up calories through exercising.

Tell your family members that if they will follow a healthy lifestyle of sensible eating and exercise, they will not have to worry about being overweight. If you have an overweight child, make sure your child knows that he or she is loved regardless of the weight. Focus on positive qualities and help the child make healthy choices, but seek professional help.

Your family may want to participate in the Presidential Sports Award. Anyone who is six years old or older can enter. There is also a Family Fitness Award for physical activity as a family. To earn the awards, participants complete activity requirements and keep a log of their activities. To learn more go to http://fitness.gov/sports/sports.html and click on the President's Sports and Fitness Award program pamphlet.

Children who are active in vigorous sports have special nutritional needs. Encourage your children to become more active, and teach them a few nutrition basics to help them perform better and protect them against injuries. For example, young athletes need to drink a lot of water, not sports drinks, and eat the right kinds of foods, not energy bars. If they are exercising hard for at least an hour, then sports drinks can replace the sodium and potassium lost through perspiration and provide carbohydrates for endurance. But in most cases, water is the best sports drink. Tell your children they should drink water before, during, and after exercise and carry a water bottle with them.

Energy bars are not a substitute for a well-balanced meal. In fact, some energy bars contain herbs and other additives that can be harmful. Energy bars will not enhance athletic ability. The calories in these bars can provide a quick burst of energy during strenuous exercise, but they are not very nutritious.

Tell the aspiring athletes in your family that they need to get enough calcium and vitamin D to keep their bones strong and less susceptible to injury. Three or four servings from the dairy food group will help provide adequate calcium and vitamin D. Discuss the following drawing for other nutritional information.

## WHAT DO NUTRIENTS DO?

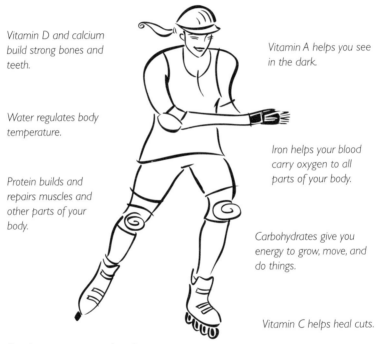

Vitamin D and calcium build strong bones and teeth.

Water regulates body temperature.

Protein builds and repairs muscles and other parts of your body.

Vitamin A helps you see in the dark.

Iron helps your blood carry oxygen to all parts of your body.

Carbohydrates give you energy to grow, move, and do things.

Vitamin C helps heal cuts.

Fat gives you energy and carries some vitamins to where they are needed.

Finally, lead everyone in a discussion of how each did on his or her individual goals for the week. Gather ideas for how to improve. Hand out certificates. (Blank certificates can be found at the end of the book—see pages 188–90.)

*Calendar for Week Four.* Show family members the calendar with week four filled out and post it where everyone can refer to it.

# ACTIVITY: RETAKE THE FITNESS TESTS

Remind everyone not to be discouraged if the test results do not show a significant positive change compared to the test results at the beginning of the thirty days. Some health improvements are not measurable right away, but assure them their bodies are healthier. Tell them that they will see a bigger difference as they continue healthy eating and exercise. Ask them if they are feeling healthier.

To do the fitness test, weigh those who participated the first time and record their weight. Repeat the flexibility test and record the furthest point reached. Next, have those who participated in the endurance test earlier do the same routine and again record the exact time in minutes and seconds. Repeat the strength test and record the number of squats. As you talk about the results, remember to give lots of praise and encouragement.

# ACTIVITY: REVIEWING HEALTHY FOODS AND GRADING NUTRITION FACT LABELS

Look at the daily values listed in percentages on the nutrition fact labels collected from various types of food. They are based on a 2000-calorie per day diet. Then look at a nutrient list: vitamins A and C, calcium, fiber, protein, and iron.

Now, make a fist.

Raise one finger for each nutrient that has 10% or more listed for its percent daily value. Keep your fingers up.

Look at the top of the label. This part lists calories and fat.

Put one finger down if either the *% daily value* of total fat is more than 10% or if there are more than 200 calories.

If you have any fingers left up, the food can be considered more nutritious. If you don't have any fingers up, the food could be considered less nutritious.

Explain to your family that this doesn't mean they can no longer eat the less nutritious foods. It means they should not eat them as often. Ask them to eat foods that leave them with two or three fingers up.

## ACTIVITY: BALLOON POP

On small slips of paper, write a "combination" food, such as a taco, burrito, omelet, chef salad, lasagna, chili, stew, hamburger, banana split, or any others you can think of. Put a slip of paper in a balloon and inflate the balloon; then tie it off. Give each family member a balloon and tell them there is something inside which they must figure out. Have them sit with the balloon underneath them and bounce up and down on the balloon until it pops. Then ask them to take out the slip of paper and read it aloud. Tell them they are supposed to name all the food groups included in the "combination" food and say whether the food is more nutritious or less nutritious. They can ask for help from other family members.

## ACTIVITY: PLAN AN ACTIVITY TO CELEBRATE EVERYONE'S ACCOMPLISHMENTS

Ask family members to brainstorm ideas for celebrating the end of the 30-day program. Activities could include going to a movie, going for a hike and picnic, going to a sporting event, or entering a 5K walk or run.

## TREAT:

**Banana Pops.** Cut a large peeled banana in half and insert a popsicle stick. Roll in granola or nuts and freeze for several hours. Serve frozen.

## NEW FOOD FOR WEEK:

**Quinoa.** Quinoa is pronounced "keen-wah." This is a grain from South America, much like white rice, but more nutritious. It even cooks faster than rice. Quinoa is a small, ivory-white, bead-shaped grain that can be used in place of rice in any dish. It has a mild taste, which makes it easy to pair with other foods and takes seasonings and sauces well. Quinoa can be found in the rice or nutrition sections of most supermarkets or in health food stores.

Quinoa is higher in protein than other grains and also contains calcium, iron, and magnesium. Protein supplies amino acids, which are the building blocks of the body. Protein also supplies energy. Calcium builds and strengthens bones. Iron carries oxygen in the blood to the body's cells and carries away the carbon dioxide. Too little iron means the red blood cells cannot carry as much oxygen, causing anemia and fatigue. Magnesium is an important part of the enzymes the body must make.

Try the recipe on the next page or make up one of your own.

## TV-FREE ACTIVITY:

Make a family time capsule in a cardboard box or a plastic storage container. Have each family member contribute something meaningful to the capsule. Spend time discussing what

## QUINOA PILAF

1 medium chopped onion
½ cup sliced mushrooms
¼ cup chopped celery
1 clove minced garlic
½ cup chopped green sweet pepper
1 tablespoon butter
1 cup quinoa
2 teaspoons bouillon granules, any flavor
2 cups water
¾ cup chopped Canadian bacon (opt.)

*Cook onion, mushrooms, celery, garlic, and green pepper in butter. Stir in quinoa, bouillon, and water. Bring mixture to a boil and reduce heat. Simmer, covered, until quinoa is tender and liquid is absorbed: 10 to 15 minutes. Add Canadian bacon (optional).*

items should be included and their significance to the family. Be sure to include a copy of a newspaper and a description of current popular culture and events. Have everyone write a short summary of the highlights in their lives so far. Put as many of the items as possible in acid-free plastic sleeves.

Children may want their own time capsules as well. Shoe boxes are a good size for individual capsules. Next, decide when the capsule is to be opened and mark the date on the container: "Do not open until ————." Select a date far enough in the future to make the contents more interesting when the capsule is opened, but not so far in the future that family members will lose interest. Five to ten years is a good time period, but let the family decide. Then pick a cool, dry place to store the capsule.

## HEALTHY HABIT:

Don't limit the family to orange juice for breakfast. Try different juices, including tomato, apple, cranberry, cranberry-orange juice mix, and pineapple. Red grape juice is an excellent choice. It is loaded with antioxidants, although it does contain a lot of sugar. Be sure any fruit drinks are labeled "100% juice."

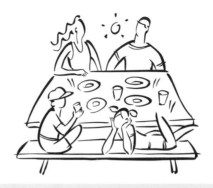

# SEASONS OF A HEALTHY FAMILY

Activities change from season to season and so do foods, offering a variety of ways for the family to become healthier. The following chapter introduces a seasonal approach that your family can use to supplement the four-week calendar.

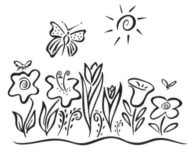

## SPRING

If your family didn't get outdoors to exercise as much as you would have liked during the winter, spring is the time to get going again. With the days getting longer, a family walk after dinner is a good start. Make it a nature walk and look for signs of spring: flowers, budding trees, insects, and birds. A pair of binoculars and field guides to trees, flowers, and birds can make the family walks even more entertaining. Field guides can be purchased or checked out from the library.

A visit to a farm or dairy farm can teach your children where their food comes from. Farms are busy, interesting places in the spring.

Spring is the time to start preparing a garden. Even a container garden can be a good family project. Have a family meeting to talk about what kind of garden to plant. Send off for seed catalogs or go to a garden center. Seed catalog Web sites include www.garden.com, www.seedrack.com, and www.gardenbazaar.com. Go as a family to your public library and check out gardening books. You will need to find out your geographic zone so you can determine which flowers and crops you can grow and how early you can plant. Most gardening books have maps that provide that information, or you can call your county or state cooperative extension office.

Spring is also the time for wonderful fruits and vegetables in season, fresh and less expensive. Watch in the grocery store or farmers' market for asparagus, green onions, peas, and strawberries.

Here are three spring recipes to try:

## CHICKEN SALAD ROLL UPS

6 whole wheat or flour tortillas

Vinaigrette:

1½ tablespoons olive oil
1½ tablespoons vinegar
1 tablespoon grainy mustard
½ teaspoon ground black pepper

Chicken Salad Filling:

3½ cups cooked, shredded chicken, loosely packed
12 large Chinese cabbage leaves, shredded
1 medium sweet red pepper, cut into very thin strips
8 green onions, sliced
4 celery stalks, sliced
1 package (about 6 ounces) alfalfa sprouts, washed thoroughly

*In a large bowl, combine all the ingredients for the filling except for the sprouts. Pour the vinaigrette over the salad and toss until blended. Set aside.*

*Place ⅙ of the chicken salad filling in a line along one side of each tortilla. Add sprouts as desired and roll up like an enchilada.*

*Serve immediately. Or, finished sandwiches can be wrapped individually in plastic and stored for up to 24 hours.*

*Nutrients per roll up:*

*Calories 330  Carbohydrate 26 g  Saturated Fat 2.6 g  Fiber 4 g  Protein 29 g  Total Fat 12 g  Cholesterol 72 mg  Sodium 317 mg*

## FROZEN FRUIT POPS (4 HOURS TO FREEZE)

1 ripe honeydew melon (optional)
2 or 3 ripe bananas
2 pints ripe strawberries
¼ cup honey or sugar

*Peel, seed, and cut fruit into chunks. Put fruit and honey or sugar in blender in small batches and puree. (Pops will taste less sweet when they are frozen.)*

*Ladle the puree into freezer pop molds and freeze for at least 4 hours or until frozen.*

*Puree can also be frozen in plastic ice cube trays. Poke wooden sticks into place when the pops are almost frozen so the sticks will stay upright.*

*Nutrients per one 2-ounce pop:*

*Calories 90  Total Fat less than 1 g  Protein 1 g  Carbohydrate 23 g  Fiber 2 g  Sodium 11 mg*

## EARLY-VEGETABLE AND LENTIL SALAD

½ cup lentils, washed
½ pound new red potatoes with skin, quartered
½ pound thin asparagus
1 cup fresh peas, shelled (in shell about ½ pound); frozen peas can be used
2 cups frozen corn
2 large carrots, shredded

Dressing:

1 tablespoon chopped, fresh parsley
1 garlic clove, finely chopped
2 tablespoons red wine vinegar

⅓ cup olive oil
1 tablespoon mustard

*Bring 1 cup water to a boil. Add the lentils and cook over low heat until tender, about 20 minutes. Drain the lentils.*

*Boil potatoes for 10–15 minutes.*

*Cut the bottom 2 inches off the asparagus. Rinse the asparagus in cold water. Remove the fresh peas from their shells.*

*Steam asparagus, peas, and corn for 3 minutes. Remove and run cold water over the vegetables to stop the cooking process.*

*For dressing: Combine the chopped parsley, chopped garlic, vinegar, and mustard in a mixing bowl. Mix together with a whisk, add the oil in a slow, steady stream.*

*Combine the lentils, potatoes, asparagus, peas, corn, and carrots. Toss with dressing. Serve.*

*Nutrients per 1 cup serving:*

*Calories 179  Saturated fat less than 1 g  Protein 6 g  Cholesterol 0  Carbohydrate 36 g  Fiber 6 g  Total Fat 5 g  Sodium 73 mg*

*(Source for all recipes in the Seasons section:* Food, Family and Fun, *U.S. Department of Agriculture, Food and Consumer Service. Used with permission.)*

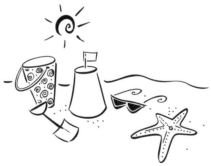

# SUMMER

Summer offers unlimited opportunities for family fitness and healthy eating. With all the fresh fruits and vegetables and the numerous exercise options, it is also a good time to lose some weight. Remember that in the summer you need to drink more water.

Plan several family hikes and take healthy snacks. Look up trails on the Internet at www.americanhiking.org. If you live in the city, take the train to a nearby recreation area or go to the park. Have a picnic, even if it's just in the backyard. The "new" experience may provide the chance for picky eaters to try different foods. Call it "special picnic food."

In early summer, go berry picking at a farm. Later in the summer you can find "pick your own" vegetable farms. Check with local farmers' markets for locations. These outdoor markets are increasingly popular and a good place to take the family. If you have a garden plot, the weeding, hoeing, and thinning can provide moderate exercise.

Riding bikes as a family is another fun activity. Bring carrot sticks, sliced apples, raisins, and other simple foods and plenty of water.

If family members like to swim, do laps in the pool.

Hold a field day and invite neighborhood families. Give out ribbons after each event. You can make your own or buy them inexpensively at a party store. To make your own, get gold foil seal stickers at an office store and cut ribbons to stick on the back. Adapt some of the events from field day at your children's school or make up some of your own. Tug of war, relay races, running and standing long jumps, sprints, hopping, cartwheels, water balloon toss, wheelbarrow races, and sack races are just a few. Try to include sports to fit each child's abilities. Very young children can ride piggy back on their parents for some of the races. Young children can run and pick up items placed in the yard and bring them back to a bucket. For another game have the younger children (or everyone) put their shoes in a pile, then see who can find their shoes and put them on in the fastest time. Brainstorm with your neighbors. Have a potluck dinner when the games are over. Another variation for your own family is to design events that center around the equipment at the local park playground. Then have a picnic.

Try planting an herb garden. It's simple. All you need is garden soil, a sunny spot, a little water, and herb seedlings. Herbs do well on a sunny window sill or in a container outside. They grow well in the ground, too. When it's time to harvest, pick the leaves in the morning just after the dew is gone and dry them in the microwave on paper towels, or in the oven, or just hang them upside down in a cool, dark place. When the leaves are dry, store them in covered glass jars in a dark place.

Nearly every fruit and vegetable you can think of is in season and reasonably priced. Apricots and cherries come earlier in the summer; plums and peaches later in the season. Tomatoes, corn on the cob, and melons are favorites, but include peppers, green beans, and summer squash in your meals too.

Some summer recipes are included below:

## WATERMELON ICE

(per person)
½ cup cracked ice
3 tablespoons sugar
Squeezed juice of 1 lime
1 cup watermelon, cubed

*Place ice, sugar, lime, and watermelon in a blender and process. Put the mixture in a freezer until slushy.*

Nutrients:

Calories 102  Sodium 3 mg  Protein 1 g  Fiber 0 g  Carbohydrate 26 g  Fat less than 1 g

## FRESH TOMATO SAUCE

3 cups chopped tomatoes
2 stems fresh oregano, chopped, or ¼ teaspoon dried oregano
1 tablespoon garlic powder
1 tablespoon onion powder

2 stems fresh parsley, chopped, or ¼ teaspoon dried parsley

2 fresh basil leaves, chopped, or ¼ teaspoon dried basil

¼ teaspoon fennel seed

⅛ teaspoon black pepper

*In a saucepan combine all sauce ingredients.*

*Simmer on medium heat for 15 minutes or until tomatoes are soft. Serve over cooked pasta.*

*Note: To remove skins from tomatoes, put them in boiling water for a few seconds. The peel will slip right off.*

*Nutrients:*

*Calories 47  Total Fat less than 1 g  Protein 2 g  Sodium 305 mg  Carbohydrate 11 g Fiber 2 g  Cholesterol 0 mg*

---

## QUICK SUMMER FRUIT SHORTCAKE

1 pint strawberries, cleaned, hulled, and quartered (or other berries)

2 peaches, diced

3 tablespoons sugar

¼ cup orange juice

4 slices angel food cake

*Combine strawberries (or other berries), peaches, sugar, and orange juice in a large bowl.*

*Mix well, cover with plastic wrap, and refrigerate for 20 minutes.*

*Top the cake with fruit mixture.*

*Nutrients:*

*Calories 148  Sodium 210 mg  Protein 2 g  Fiber 2 g  Carbohydrate 36 g  Cholesterol 0 mg  Total Fat Less than 1 g*

---

## MIXED BERRY CRISP

1 cup flour

½ cup sugar

1 teaspoon cinnamon

4 tablespoons butter

6 cups mixed fresh or frozen berries, thawed (blueberries, straw-
    berries, raspberries, and blackberries)

*Combine flour, sugar, and cinnamon in a bowl; blend in butter until mixture is crumbly. Place berries in non-stick baking dish and sprinkle crumb mixture over them. Bake at 375° F for 20 to 30 minutes.*

Source: 5-a-Day Association of Utah

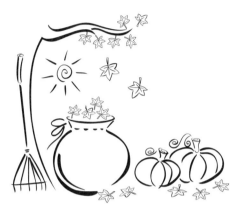

# FALL

Fall is back-to-school time, and finding time for family exercise becomes a challenge. At this time of year, hikes, bike rides, and other outside activities can be even more pleasant than during the warmer months. Take advantage of the beauty of autumn and the crisp, cool air to rake leaves or collect leaves. When the family has collected some beautiful specimens, dry them between pages of the phone book or in a flower press. When the leaves are completely dry, your family can make beautiful coasters. Here's how.

Have pieces of clear glass cut three to three-and-a-half inches square and one-eighth inch thick. Ask the glass cutter to sand the edges. You will need two pieces of glass for each coaster. You will also need a roll of copper foil tape, one-quarter inch thick. You can get foil tape at stores that make decorative window glass. Place a leaf or leaves in the center of the glass (do not overlap) and cover them with the other glass square. Secure the glass while you work by using clips. Remove the adhesive backing from the copper tape as you cover the edges of the glass "sandwich" with the foil. Press the foil firmly to the glass. These coasters make lovely gifts.

Fall is harvest time. The supermarkets and farmers' markets are stocked with summer fruits and vegetables, and, as October arrives, winter squash and pumpkins abound. Fall apples, potatoes, and sweet potatoes also become available. Find out if apple picking is available in your area. Have an apple-tasting party. Buy several varieties of apples and cut them into wedges. Label each plate of sliced apples with the name of the variety. Let everyone try each variety and pick favorites. You can even throw a little math in by graphing the results. Apples can be stored for months in the refrigerator if you place them in plastic zip bags and keep them as far to the back of the refrigerator as possible, where it is the coldest.

Recipes which take advantage of fall's bounty are included below.

## PORK CHOPS WITH APPLES

4 small apples (Macintosh apples have a sweet taste. For tartness, use Granny Smith)
vegetable oil spray
4 pork chops, ½ inch thick, trimmed of all fat
¼ teaspoon salt and ⅛ teaspoon pepper
1 tablespoon vegetable oil

*Core apples and cut into quarters. Then cut each quarter into 3 or 4 slices.*

*Spray a skillet with vegetable spray and heat over medium heat. Brown chops on both sides for 3–5 minutes. Salt and pepper the pork chops.*

*Push pork chops to the center of the skillet. Place apples around chops. Drizzle oil over the top of apples. Cook for 5 minutes, shaking the pan from time to time and turning the apple slices over to brown both sides.*

*Remove chops from pan to a serving plate and surround with the apples.*

*Nutrients:*

*Calories 250  Cholesterol 52 mg  Protein 19 g  Sodium 42 mg  Carbohydrate 21 g Fiber 4 g  Total fat 10.4 g  Saturated fat 3 g*

# HARVEST PUMPKIN BREAD

1 cup sugar

¼ cup margarine

¼ cup applesauce

2 eggs

1 cup (8 oz) solid-pack pumpkin

2 cups all-purpose flour

½ teaspoon salt

2 teaspoons baking powder

¼ teaspoon baking soda

1 teaspoon ground cinnamon

½ cup raisins

1 teaspoon grated orange rind

¼ cup orange juice

½ cup chopped walnuts (optional)

*Preheat oven to 350° F.*

*Lightly grease a 9" x 5" x 3" loaf pan or coat it with vegetable spray.*

*Beat sugar, margarine, and applesauce until creamy and light (about 5 minutes).*

*Add eggs one at a time and continue to beat.  Add pumpkin and mix until smooth.*

*Combine flour, salt, baking powder, baking soda, and cinnamon. Stir into pumpkin mixture and mix until smooth.*

*Add raisins, orange rind, orange juice, and nuts. Stir well, then pour the mixture into the loaf pan.*

*Bake at 350° F. for 60 to 65 minutes.  Test doneness by sticking a wooden pick into the loaf. If it comes out clean, the loaf is done.*

*Nutrients:*

*Calories 220 per slice, 12 slices per loaf  Cholesterol 35 mg  Protein 4 g  Sodium 261 mg  Carbohydrate 42 g  Fiber 2 g  Total fat 5 g  Saturated fat 1 g*

## STUFFED POTATOES

*Bake potatoes in the oven or save time by cooking them in the microwave.*

4 large potatoes
1 tablespoon oil
4 tablespoons grated lowfat cheese (mozzarella or cheddar)
¼ teaspoon salt
⅛ teaspoon pepper
⅛ teaspoon nutmeg

*Preheat oven to 425° F. Scrub potatoes well. Dry with a paper towel and rub the outside with oil. Bake until the potatoes are soft, about 45 to 60 minutes.*

*Cut off a potato cap lengthwise. Scoop out some of the potato and mix with the cheese, salt, pepper, and nutmeg. Spoon the mixture back into the potato. Replace the cap and serve.*

*Vary the toppings by using leftover meat, mashed beans, cooked broccoli, or other toppings your family likes.*

*Nutrients: (basic recipe)*

*Calories 262  Cholesterol 1 mg  Protein 6 g  Sodium 204 mg  Total fat 4 g  Fiber 5 g Saturated fat 1 g*

---

## SWEET POTATO SMASHIES

1 large sweet potato
1 egg, lightly beaten
2 teaspoons vegetable cooking oil
nonstick cooking spray
⅔ cup flour
¼ cup packed brown sugar
½ teaspoon baking powder
¼ teaspoon baking soda
¾ cup golden raisins or dried, chopped apricots
1½ teaspoons ground cinnamon
dried raisins or chopped dates for decorating

*Pierce sweet potato three times with fork. Cook sweet potato in microwave on HIGH about 5 minutes or until tender when pierced with a fork.*

*When sweet potato is cool enough to handle, cut open and scoop out ½ cup; then combine sweet potato, egg, and oil in a small bowl.*

*Preheat oven to 375° F. Lightly coat a baking sheet with cooking spray.*

*Combine flour, sugar, baking powder, baking soda, golden raisins or chopped apricots, and cinnamon in a medium bowl; set aside.*

*Add sweet potato mixture to flour mixture. Stir until thoroughly combined.*

*Spoon mixture, two tablespoons at a time, onto baking sheet to make 8 mounds.*

*Moisten fingertips with water and smash mounds gently with fingertips to about ½ inch thickness. Arrange raisins or chopped dates to make eyes, nose, and mouth.*

*Bake for 15 minutes or until very lightly browned and smashies spring back when lightly touched. Remove baking tray from oven. With pancake turner, remove from baking sheets and cool on wire rack.*

*Source: California 5-a-Day.*

# WINTER

Winter does not have to be a season of inactivity. In areas where winter weather is cold, winter sports like snowshoeing, skiing, sledding, cross-country skiing, and ice skating are all good forms of exercise. But even if these activities are not available, winter can still provide opportunities to be physically fit. Snow shoveling is a good family activity. Get the neighborhood together and shovel the drives and walkways of elderly or sick neighbors; when you're finished, get together for hot chocolate.

Many communities have public indoor pools where the family can swim together for exercise. Some high schools have indoor tracks for jogging and walking, or dress properly and take brisk walks outside.

Winter is a good time to start a family, extended family, or neighborhood newspaper. In addition to providing a TV-free activity, children learn how to interview, write, and compose a "newspaper." The newspaper can easily be prepared on the computer. School credit might even be available. Take the family to the local newspaper office and get ideas. See if local businesses want to advertise.

Another fun winter activity is searching your family history. Check out Web sites like www.familysearch.org (free), www.genealogy.com, or www.myfamily.com to get started. Try spending some winter evenings finding out about your ancestors.

Gardening is another winter activity! Artificial lights, soil-less potting mixes, and shelves are all the materials needed to grow plants during the winter. Good advice on winter gardens can be found at www.agweb.okstate.edu. Click on "PEARL," then "horticulture," and go to "gardening for kids."

There are still many seasonal foods available in the winter, like citrus fruits. Oranges are inexpensive this time of year. Get a bag full of oranges and a plastic juicer, and let the children squeeze their own orange juice.

Winter pears, sweet potatoes, carrots, cabbage, broccoli, brussels sprouts, winter squash, and cauliflower are in peak season during the cold weather months. Apples harvested in the fall are also available at good prices.

Winter can bring out the "nesting instinct" in people. Perhaps that is why some people enjoy baking and cooking this time of year. Hot cereal is nutritious and especially welcome in the winter. When making hot cereal like oatmeal, put in raisins and try adding applesauce or canned peaches as a topping instead of sugar. Hearty soups are also a winter favorite.

Some winter recipes are:

## CARROT BARS

1 cup sugar
½ cup vegetable oil
¼ cup applesauce
2 small jars baby food carrots
2 eggs, beaten
1¼ cup flour
1 teaspoon vanilla
1 teaspoon baking soda
1 teaspoon cinnamon
½ teaspoon salt
½ cup nuts, chopped (optional)
Powdered sugar

*Preheat oven to 350° F. Mix sugar, oil, applesauce, baby food carrots, eggs, flour, vanilla, baking soda, cinnamon, salt, and nuts together.*
*Bake in 9" x 13" greased and floured pan for 25 to 30 minutes.*
*When bars are cool, sprinkle with powdered sugar and cut into bars.*

*Nutrients:*

*Calories 71   Sodium 73 mg   Protein 1 g   Fiber 0 g   Carbohydrate 10 g   Cholesterol 11 mg   Total fat 3 g   Saturated fat 1/2 g*

## NEW OATMEAL RAISIN COOKIES

¾ cup sugar
2 tablespoon margarine or butter
1 large egg
2 tablespoons low-fat or skim milk
¼ cup applesauce
¾ cup all-purpose flour
¼ teaspoon baking soda
½ teaspoon ground cinnamon
⅛ teaspoon ground nutmeg
¼ teaspoon salt

1¼ cups quick oats
½ cup raisins

*Preheat oven to 350° F.*

*On medium speed, cream sugar and margarine or butter until smooth and creamy.*

*Add egg and mix on medium speed for one minute.*

*Add milk and applesauce and mix for one more minute. Scrape the sides of the bowl.*

*In a small bowl, combine flour, baking soda, cinnamon, nutmeg, and salt. Add dry ingredients to the creamed mixture and mix on low speed for two minutes until blended.*

*Add oats and raisins and blend for 30 seconds on low speed. Scrape the sides of the bowl.*

*Drop dough by rounded teaspoons onto lightly greased cookie sheets.*

*Bake for 10 to 13 minutes until lightly browned. Cool on a wire rack.*

Nutrients:

Calories 70　Cholesterol 8 mg　Protein 1 g　Sodium 42 mg　Carbohydrate 14 g　Fiber 1 g　Total fat 1 g　Saturated fat less than 1 g

---

## HEARTY VEGETABLE SOUP

1½ cups water

1 quart vegetable or chicken broth—low fat, low sodium

1 can pinto or kidney beans (or soak 1½ tablespoons dry pinto beans overnight in 1 cup cold water covered, in the refrigerator. In the morning, discard the water, and rinse the beans.)

2 tablespoons dry lentils

¼ cup pearled barley

¼ cup onions, diced

½ cup fresh carrots, diced

¼ cup fresh celery, diced

½ cup fresh white potatoes, peeled and cubed

1 tablespoon tomato paste

½ teaspoon pepper

½ cup frozen corn

½ cup frozen cut green beans

½ cup fresh cabbage, shredded

*In a large saucepan, bring 1½ cups water and broth to a boil.*

*Add soaked pinto beans, lentils, barley, onions, carrots, celery, potatoes, tomato paste, and pepper. Cover and simmer for 20 minutes.*

*Add corn, green beans, and cabbage. Simmer, covered, for 15 minutes. Note: If using canned beans, add them at this stage.*

*Nutrients:*

*Calories 122  Sodium 65 mg (more if using canned beans)  Protein 8 g   Carbohydrate 21 g  Fiber 5 g  Total Fat 1 g  Cholesterol 0 mg*

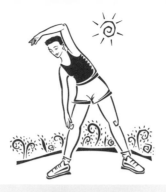

# EXERCISE

*Get your doctor's OK before starting your family on an aerobic or strength training program.* Strength training can begin as early as seven years old, if performed properly. The following exercises can be done as a family. Younger children can do them with or without weights or bands. If an exercise is not advised for children, it is noted. Some exercises for children younger than seven years old are provided.

For those who want to lose weight, keep in mind that dieting without strength training can cause fat loss *and* muscle loss. Sustained weight loss and weight management requires strength training. Exercise builds lean muscle mass. The larger the lean muscle mass, the more calories the body burns. (It is not necessary to use protein supplements. A healthy eating plan provides more than enough protein for muscle building.)

The following exercises require several sets of dumbbells: three-pound, five-pound, and eight-pound. Heavier weights can be added later, if needed. The exercises also require some surgical tubing or exercise bands. Surgical tubing and exercise bands can be purchased inexpensively at a medical supply store. Buy bands in different tensions. Change the tension of bands and surgical tubing by making them shorter or longer. Buy two two-foot lengths of tubing. A couple of other useful and inexpensive pieces of exercise equipment include a

## FITNESS TIPS AT YOUR DESK

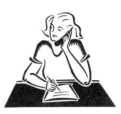

- Stretch throughout the day.
  It is a vital part of exercise.

- Squeeze a tennis ball to help
  strengthen your hand and wrist.

- Using a chair to brace yourself,
  do some calf raises to increase
  muscle strength.

- How about using that speakerphone. Did you know
  that more calories are burned while standing?

- Shoulder rolls: forward ten times, then repeat
  circling backward.

- While sitting at your desk, rotate one foot to "write"
  each letter of the alphabet. Switch feet and repeat.

- Wall sits: stand with back against wall. Slowly lower
  into a sitting position. Hold for 30 seconds. Repeat.

- Get out of your chair and move around for a few
  minutes every hour.

- Shoulder shrugs are a great way to loosen up tight
  muscles. Repeat 5 to 10 times.

- Keep a water cup close by, but don't forget to get
  up and fill it up. Everyone should drink eight
  8-ounce glasses of water each day.

- Stretch your lower back. While seated, slowly bend
  forward at the waist. Reach forward with your
  hands until they touch the floor. Hold for 15 seconds before slowly coming up.

- Move your feet and legs while you're sitting at your
  desk to burn calories and increase energy.

(From the Utah Department of Health Cardiovascular Program.
Used by permission.)

large exercise ball, which can be found at a sporting goods store, and a child's ball, about six inches in diameter. For a change from the exercises in this book, rent or buy strength training videos. Rent some first to try them out. Do not rely on just one video, however, because muscles adapt to the same exercises after a few weeks and results will diminish. Muscles need to be challenged.

The strength and toning exercises listed here can be done twice a week, but not more than three times a week if you are doing all of them—upper body and lower body—at once. Muscles need days off to repair themselves. This is true for all but the stomach exercises and the thigh exercises that are done without bands or weights. These can be done daily, if you want. Another option is to alternate days by doing upper body exercises one day and lower body exercises the next. Choose whichever system is most convenient for you and your family.

Most of the exercises here consist of two to three sets of eight to twelve repetitions (reps) each. When you are no longer fatigued at twelve reps, you can add more sets or do more reps. When using weights, increase the weight whenever you feel ready, and continue to do so, until you reach the limit that you can lift. Lifting heavier weights in fewer repetitions is called the overload principle and is an effective way for adults to build muscle.

## Strength and Toning Exercises

Do not do all of the exercises at once—there are enough so you can switch them around every week or so. Pick upper body, stomach, and lower body exercises and do a total of eight sets (from eight to fifteen reps per set) each session. If you cannot do eight reps, the weight you are using is too heavy. The last rep should be difficult. Keep in mind that you should not work more than two or three muscle groups per exercise session. Make each movement slow and controlled. Exhale on the exertion stage of the exercise and inhale on the recovery stage. Keep the stomach muscles firm. Any of the band exercises can be done with tubing instead.

# UPPER BODY EXERCISES

## CHEST PRESS WITH BAND

1. Place the band around the upper back and under the armpits.

2. Hold on to the ends of the band and adjust the length by wrapping it around the hands to get the 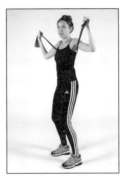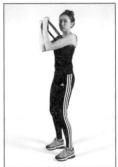 desired tension. Keep the elbows bent with the hands at forehead height and press the elbows into the center of the body.

3. Return to the starting position. Do eight to ten, rest, and repeat if you can.

## EXTENDED CHEST PRESS WITH BAND

1. Place the band around the upper back and under the armpits.

2. Keep arms straight, and move the hands towards each other so they meet in front of the 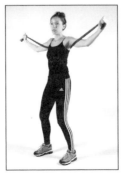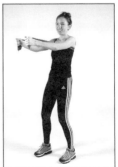 chest, arms extended. Do eight to ten, rest, and try to repeat.

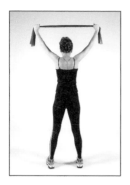 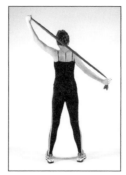 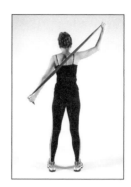

## LAT PULL DOWNS

1. Hold the ends of the band in each hand, over your head. Keep the tension as tight as possible.

2. Lower first one arm and then the other behind the head, elbows slightly bent until you have stretched as far down as possible.

3. Slowly raise each arm again back over the head. Do ten to fifteen reps, rest, and repeat.

## SEATED ROW

1. Sit with your legs extended in front of you.

2. Hook the band around the soles of your feet, holding each end with your hands at knee level.

3. Pull the ends of the band towards you with your elbows close to your sides and your back straight.

4. Slowly return to starting position. Do fifteen reps, rest, and repeat.

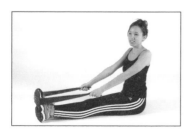 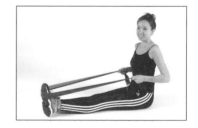

## SHOULDER PRESS

1. Standing with feet shoulder-width apart and knees slightly bent, take dumbbells (start out light if you need to) with both hands.

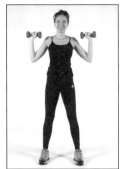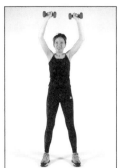

2. With palms facing forward and elbows all the way down, lift the dumbbells slowly straight up over your head, pausing at ear level.

3. Return slowly. Do fifteen times and repeat.

## BICEPS CURLS

1. In standing position, hold dumb-bells at sides with palms facing forward.

2. Slowly curl up dumbbells to chest level.

3. Return to start-ing position, slow

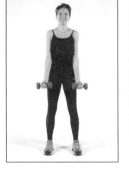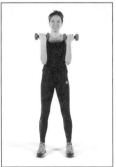

and controlled. Do fifteen reps and repeat if you can.

## CHEST FLY

1. Lie on back on ball to get the full range of motion with your arms. Have knees bent, feet flat on the floor.

2. Take dumbbells and extend arms, elbows slightly bent.

3. Move arms overhead until hands are two inches apart.

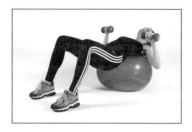
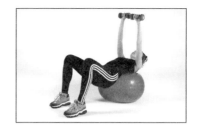

4. Lower arms with elbows bent until upper arms are as close to the floor as possible. Do fifteen times and repeat if possible.

## MODIFIED PUSH-UP (NOT FOR KIDS)

1. Get on hands and knees, with hands shoulder-width apart, fingers pointing forward.

2. Lift calves off the floor and cross ankles.

3. Lower body toward floor until elbows are at a 90-degree angle. Keep back flat.

4. Push straight up. Repeat as many times as possible. The first thing to touch the floor should be your nose, not your thighs. You should be on the upper part of the knee, not the kneecap. If these are too difficult, you can try doing standing push-ups against a wall at first.

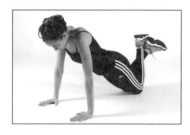
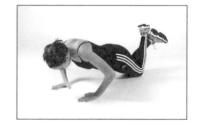

## CHAIR DIP (NOT FOR KIDS)

1. Sit on the edge of a chair with legs extended and hands holding onto the seat alongside your hips.

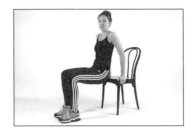 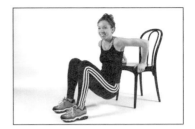

2. Keeping your arms straight, slide your bottom off the chair and bend the knees slightly so your feet are flat on the floor.

3. Lower your body, bending the elbows until the upper arms are parallel to the floor.

4. Pause and slowly push yourself back up. These are difficult. Do as many as possible, working up to ten times. Remember to keep your body close to the chair.

## TRICEPS EXTENSION

1. Stand with back straight and knees slightly bent.

2. Hold a three- to five-pound dumbbell with both hands and raise it over your head, elbows in close.

3. Relax, and let

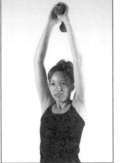 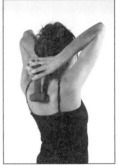

the weight dangle towards the floor behind your head.

4. Keeping arms close to your head and bending the elbows, lower the weight behind your head as far as you can.

5. Pause, and lift the weight slowly back up. Repeat as many times as possible, working up to twenty reps. Be sure to keep your elbows close to your ears at all times.

## TRICEPS KICKBACK

1. Bend at the waist, with your elbows bent 90 degrees.

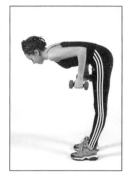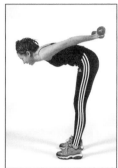

2. Hold a three- to five-pound dumbbell in each hand. Keep shoulders relaxed and elbows close to your body.

3. Point your palms inward, hands in front of your hips.

4. From the elbow, move your arms straight behind you and rotate your palms so they face upward. Keep upper arms still. Repeat up to ten times.

## LYING FRENCH PRESS

1. Lie on your back with knees bent and feet flat on floor.

2. With palms facing the floor, take a bar or dumbbells (keeping them even) and raise them until your hands are over your shoulders, elbows relaxed.

3. Keeping your upper arms still, slowly lower the bar or dumbbells toward your head, until arms are at right angles.

4. Return until your hands are over your shoulders again. Repeat ten to fifteen times. Do two more sets.

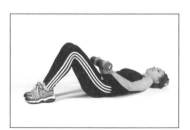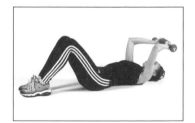

## STRETCHES

Do this after each exercise session.

1. Stand tall and roll your shoulders back several times.

2. Roll shoulders forward several times.

3. Take your left arm straight across your upper body and push it toward the chest with your right arm.

4. Repeat with the other arm.

# ABDOMINALS

Abdominals can be done every day. When doing them, always exhale as you sit up and inhale as you lie back down.

## CRUNCH

Do up to three sets of eight to twelve reps.

1. Lie on a mat or towel, eyes facing the ceiling, fingertips behind your head, elbows out. Have knees bent, feet flat on the floor.

2. Using your stomach muscles (abs), lift your head and shoulder blades off the floor, but keep your lower back on the floor. Do not pull up with your head. Take three seconds to curl up.

3. Hold for three seconds.

4. Take three seconds to curl back down.

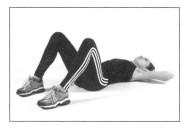 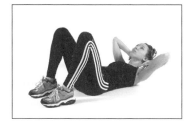

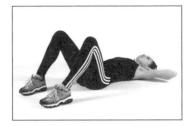 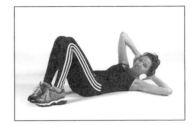

## OBLIQUE CRUNCH

1. Lie on a mat or towel, eyes facing the ceiling, hands lightly touching the sides of your head.

2. As you slowly curl your head and shoulders off the floor, twist your upper body so your right elbow is pointing toward your left knee. Lie back down, then curl your head and shoulders off the floor again, twisting to the right so your left elbow is pointing toward your right knee. Alternate from side to side as many times as you can.

## REVERSE CRUNCH

1. Lie flat on your back, arms straight down at the sides.

2. Lift your knees so your shins are parallel to the floor.

3. Slowly curl knees toward your chest, pressing your lower back into the floor.

4. Slowly lower until shins are parallel to the floor again. Repeat for one minute.

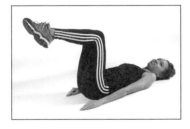 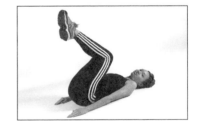

## STRETCHES

1. Lie on your back, legs out straight, and feet pointed. Arms should be straight behind you, close to your head.

2. Simultaneously stretch your legs toward your toes and your arms toward fingertips. Hold for 30 seconds.

3. Turn over so you are face down on the floor with your arms extended in front of you.

4. Lift your right leg and your left arm.

5. Hold the stretch, then lower.

6. Switch sides and repeat.

# LOWER BODY EXERCISES

Just a few notes before you get started. Do not do pliés, squats, or lunges if you have knee problems. Pay attention to your breathing: Exhale on exertion, inhale on recovery. Move slowly and deliberately. Keep stomach tight. Any of the band exercises can be done with tubing instead.

## PLIÉS

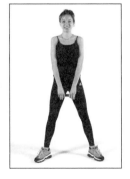 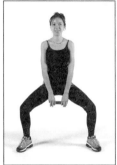

1. Stand with feet a little more than shoulder-width apart, toes pointing out, and knees slightly bent.

2. Hold a dumbbell with both hands between legs.

3. Bend your knees until they are at a 90-degree angle. Keep your back straight; knees should not go beyond toes—you should be able to see your toes, otherwise the position is wrong.

4. Return to starting position. Try this exercise first without weight, holding onto a chair for balance.

## SQUAT

It is important in this exercise to have proper form, which is why the large exercise ball is useful. When there is not enough time for several lower-body exercises, do this one instead. It can be done with or without the weights.

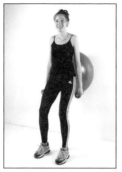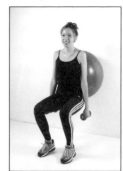

1. Start in a standing position, feet shoulder-width apart. Your weight should be on your heels and the ball should be between the wall and your back.

2. Hold the dumbbells in each hand at mid-thigh; do not push back into the wall. Use as much weight as possible, without pushing back into the wall.

3. Roll down the wall until you are in a seated position, with knees at 90 degrees.

4. Roll back up. Do two or three sets of up to twenty reps each.

## LUNGE (NOT FOR KIDS)

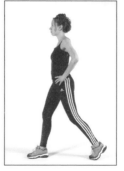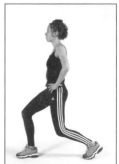

1. Stand straight, feet shoulder-width apart, with hands on hips.

2. Take a long step forward with your right foot. It should be flat on the floor. Your left foot should be on its ball.

3. Bend your left knee and lower your body, looking straight ahead with your body upright. Steps two and three are done in one motion.

4. Return to the starting position. Remember that your support leg knee should never extend past your toe. Repeat up to fifteen times on each leg.

## REVERSE LUNGE (NOT FOR KIDS)

1. Stand straight, feet shoulder-width apart, with your hands on your hips.

2. Keeping your left leg straight, step back with your left foot as far as possible.

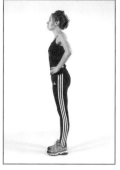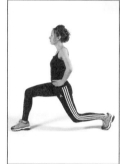

3. Lower your left knee as low as you can. Your right knee should be bent at a 90-degree angle. Steps two and three are done in one motion.

4. Lift yourself back to the starting position, tightening your bottom. Repeat ten times and then do the same with your right leg.

## SIDE LEG RAISES WITH BAND

1. Tie the band around your thighs just above the knees. The band should be tight enough to feel the resistance.

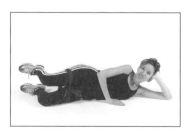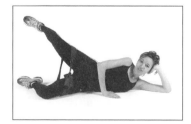

2. Lie on one side with knees bent and heels lined up with your bottom. Be sure to keep your toes and knees facing forward.

3. Slowly raise and lower the upper leg, keeping knee in line with foot. Do two sets of fifteen reps. Repeat with other leg.

## KNEE PRESS WITH BAND

1. Sit down and tie band across your knees.

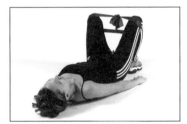

2. Lie down on your back on a mat or towel with your knees bent and your feet together, flat on the floor.

3. Press against the band by pushing outward with your knees.

4. Pause, then bring knees together. Remember to keep your pelvis up. Do up to three sets of fifteen reps, resting a few seconds between sets.

## HAMSTRING BALL

1. Get on elbows and knees, with ball or a five-pound weight behind your left knee, elbows under shoulders.

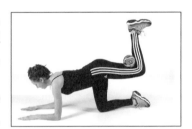

2. Lift your left leg to hip level. Keep your back straight, stomach tight. Do not twist your hips.

3. Pulse leg up and down, foot flexed, with ball in position. This is a small movement.

4. Switch legs and repeat. Do each leg up to twenty times.

## QUAD LIFT

The following thigh exer-
cises can be done with or without a band or tubing. Or use
ankle weights instead of a band
or tubing. Do these every day
without weights, or every other
day with weights or bands.

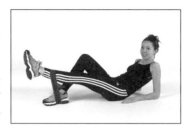

1. Tie the ends of the band together, with less tension at
first—adjust tension as you progress.

2. Lie back, one foot flat on floor, the other extended in
front of your body, resting on your elbows with lower back
pressed to ground.

3. Loop the band around one ankle and hold it down with
the other foot, as shown.

4. Slowly lift straight leg up as high as opposite knee.

5. Return to starting position and repeat, doing three sets
of fifteen reps. Repeat with the other leg.

## KNEE EXTENSIONS

1. Tie ends of band together.

2. Sit up straight on a chair or bench, one foot flat on floor,
the other leg bent and lifted toward chest.

3. Loop the band around one ankle and hold it down with
the other foot.

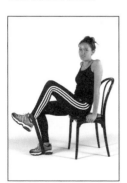
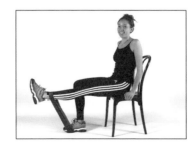

4. Slowly straighten the knee without dropping the leg, but do not lock the knee.

5. Return to starting position and repeat, doing three sets of fifteen reps. Repeat with other leg.

## BOTTOM LIFT

1. Lie on your stomach, one knee bent with ankle flexed, and heel toward your bottom.

2. Put the band on the foot of the flexed leg and around your ankle on the anchor leg.

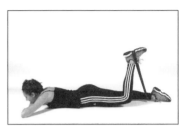

3. Tighten your bottom. Lift the bent leg slightly off the ground, and press your flexed foot toward the ceiling. Do not arch your back. Keep hips on the ground.

4. Return to starting position and repeat, doing three sets of ten to fifteen reps, if possible. Repeat with the other leg.

## HAMSTRING CURL

1. Lie on your stomach, tightening your bottom.

2. Bend one knee to lift your leg slightly off the ground. Put the band around your ankle on the curling leg and around your foot on the anchor leg.

3. While holding this position, slowly curl your heel toward your bottom. Keep your hips on the ground and do not arch your back.

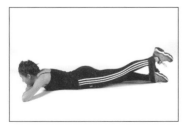
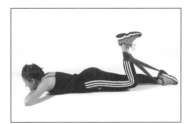

4. Return to starting position and repeat, doing three sets of ten to fifteen reps. Repeat with other leg.

## THIGH LIFT

1. Lie on your side, with your head resting on your arm.

2. Your top leg should be bent and resting on the floor in front of your bottom leg, which is bent slightly. You can put a band around your thighs or ankles to increase intensity.

3. Lift bottom leg, tightening your inner thigh. Continue lifting then lowering bottom leg without touching the ground. Be sure your hips and knees are forward. Repeat fifteen times, turn over and do the other leg.

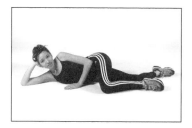 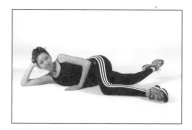

## STRETCHES

1. Get on your hands and knees and arch your back up.

2. Hold the stretch.

3. Sink your back down and hold the stretch. Repeat several times.

4. Sit on the floor with legs outstretched.

5. Pull one knee toward your chest and hug it, holding the stretch. Repeat with other leg.

6. Sit on the floor with your legs out straight.

7. Bend over slowly, sliding your right hand past your right knee, towards your feet. Reach until you feel the stretch; don't bounce. Pause and repeat with left leg.

8. This stretch can also be done using a bench. Stand, put one leg straight out on the bench, lean forward and stretch, repeat with other leg.

## Aerobic Exercise

The word *aerobic* means "with oxygen." An aerobic exercise is one in which the large muscles of the body (arms and legs) move in continuous, rhythmical motion, raising the heart rate to between 60 percent and 90 percent of the maximum heart rate. This rate is the maximum number of beats per minute that the heart can attain. To estimate this rate, subtract your age from 220. For example, if you are 45 years old, you have a maximum heart rate of 175 beats per minute. You should exercise at a pace that keeps your heart rate between 105 and 157 beats per minute. This is your aerobic training range. In this range, carbohydrates *and fats* are burned, and oxygen reaches the muscles, where it is converted to muscular energy. If, when you are exercising, you are breathing hard but still can carry on a conversation, you know you are in your aerobic range. If you are out of breath and cannot talk, your exercise will not be as effective and you may experience more muscle soreness. In addition, you will not be able to keep up the pace long enough to burn fat as an energy source. However, a faster pace on some days can provide additional health benefits besides weight loss. Researchers have found that vigorous exercise reduces the risk of heart disease more than exercising at a more moderate rate. Exercise in general will lower cholesterol, lower high blood pressure, protect against diabetes, and fight heart disease.

To find your heart rate while exercising, stop briefly and find your pulse. Then, starting from zero, count the number of heartbeats for ten seconds and multiply that number by six to find your heart rate per minute. (This needs to be done quickly because your pulse will drop rapidly.) A heart rate monitor which straps around the chest is a convenient but costly way to help you stay within your aerobic range. The monitors can be purchased from a sporting goods store for about $80 to $100.

Brisk walking, running, jogging, swimming, skating, bicycling, rowing, cross-country skiing, and jump roping are all examples of aerobic activities. Fitness experts suggest *at least* 30 minutes of aerobic exercise, five days a week. To see better results in terms of weight loss, 60 minutes per day, five days a week is the latest recommendation. The exercise does not have to be done all at one time. If breaking up the 30 to 60 minutes into shorter exercise sessions throughout the day is more convenient, it is still as effective. (It is better to eat *after* exercising, when your metabolism is elevated. If that is not possible, wait thirty minutes after eating to allow your food to settle before you exercise.)

*If your family is new to exercise, start off slowly* and work up to the recommended amount. Any exercise is better than none at all. The more aerobically fit your family members become, the less tired they will feel and the better they will sleep. Studies also show that fit individuals are happier. Explain to your family that as they exercise, their heart muscles are strengthened, enabling the heart to pump more blood with each beat. This in turn makes it possible for the heart to beat less often to supply the same amount of blood to the body. This means the heart will last longer.

## WARM UP

Always warm up and stretch before beginning aerobic exercise. Afterwards, cool down and stretch again. Warm up or cool down by slowing the intensity of the workout for about five to ten minutes. Stretch **hamstrings** by standing on one leg and propping the other leg parallel to the ground on a bench or other raised surface. Bend over and slide your hands toward the propped-up ankle as far as they will go, but do not bounce. Repeat with the other leg. The **quadriceps** stretch is done by putting your left hand on a wall or tree for balance, then reaching behind the back with the right hand and grabbing the ankle of the right leg. Pull it up toward your bottom until you can feel the stretch in the front of your thigh. Repeat on the opposite side. Stretch the **Achilles tendon** and **calf muscles** by placing both hands against a wall or tree. Place one foot way behind you. Keep the rear leg straight with its heel on the ground and lean in toward the wall or tree. Repeat with the other leg.

## GETTING STARTED

One of the easiest and least expensive ways to get an aerobic workout is by walking briskly. Good walking shoes are the only requirement. To find out how your aerobic fitness is progressing, measure off a four-mile distance in your car. Then walk it, keeping within your aerobic range, and see how long it takes. About every four or five weeks, walk that route again and see if you can finish it faster each time, still staying within your aerobic range. Work towards completing a mile in 15 to 20 minutes. Walking at a rate of four miles per hour burns 492 calories in one hour. On some days, pick up your pace and jog. Your body will soon get used to the same walk and the benefits from it will begin to diminish. The body gets conditioned to certain intensities, thus necessitating an increase. To do this, change the exercise a little. For example, take a new route that includes hills, raise your arms above

```
..........................................................
. ┌──────────────────────────────────────────────┐ .
.                    TAKE A BREAK                    .
.                                                    .
. ❧ Spice up your breaks with a jaunt around the build- .
.     ing.                                            .
. ❧ Do you need to clear your head? Get up and take a .
.     five-minute walk.                               .
. ❧ If you can't take a break to walk for 20 minutes, try .
.     taking two 10-minute breaks.                    .
. ❧ Leave a few minutes early for meetings to allow   .
.     time to stretch your legs a bit.                .
. ❧ Using the phone to talk to the person down the    .
.     hall? Get up and get moving. The walk will do you .
.     good.                                           .
. ❧ Top off your lunch hour with a 15-minute          .
.     walk.                                           .
. ❧ Going out to lunch? Why not                       .
.     choose a spot some distance away                .
.     and walk.                                       .
. ❧ Eat some carbohydrates, fruits,                   .
.     and vegetables for energy.                      .
.                                                     .
.     (From the Utah Department of Health             .
.     Cardiovascular Program. Used by permission.)    .
..........................................................
```

your head or at heart level while you are walking, or walk on an unpaved road instead of a paved road. You can also intersperse a walk with periods of more speed. For example, walk three blocks, then jog one block. Drink plenty of water before, during, and after exercise.

Make exercise part of your family's time together. *Always wear protective gear:* helmet, knee pads, and so on, depending on the exercise. Plan activities like you plan your meals. Swimming is a good family activity, as are walks, bicycling, and hikes. As a game, time your family walks and try to beat your previous time. Another idea is to fill an activity box with different types of exercise and sports listed on slips of paper. Once a week someone may draw an activity from the box, which then becomes the family's exercise for that week. Participate as a family in the Presidential Sports Award program, which is sponsored by the President's Council on Physical Fitness and Sports and the Amateur Athletic Union. Anyone over six years of age is eligible. To find out more you can write to the Presidential Sports Award, c/o Walt Disney World Resort, P.O. Box 10000, Lake Buena Vista, FL 32839-1000. Telephone 407-934-7200. Fax 407-934-7242.

Most importantly, have fun!

## FITNESS TIPS FOR GETTING TO WORK

❧ Ride your bicycle to work.

❧ Get off the bus a few stops from your work and walk the rest of the way.

❧ Park your car as far away as possible and allow extra time to walk to work.

❧ Come to work ½ hour early or stay after to jog or walk.

❧ Try taking the stairs instead of the elevator. At first you may want to ride the elevator halfway before starting your climb. Add more floors as you increase your energy.

(From the Utah Department of Health Cardiovascular Program. Used by permission.)

# Activity Record

| | ACTIVITY | INTENSITY | MON | TUES | WED | THU | FRI | SAT |
|---|---|---|---|---|---|---|---|---|
| | | | FREQUENCY & DURATION | | | | | |
| Example: | jogging | moderate | 25 | 30 | | 20 | | |
| | | | | | | | | |
| | | | | | | | | |
| | | | | | | | | |
| | | | | | | | | |
| | | | | | | | | |
| | | | | | | | | |
| | | | | | | | | |
| | | | | | | | | |
| | | | | | | | | |
| | | | | | | | | |
| | | | | | | | | |
| | | | | | | | | |
| | | | | | | | | |
| | | | | | | | | |
| | | | | | | | | |
| | | | | | | | | |
| | | | | | | | | |
| | | | | | | | | |
| | | | | | | | | |
| | | | | | | | | |

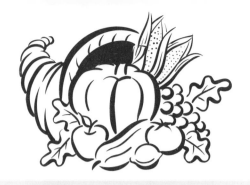

# HEALTHY FOODS

Having healthy foods available for yourself and your family will make it easier for all of you to eat sensibly. Post a list of suggested snacks from the foods you have on hand on the refrigerator. A healthy snack can also make a good breakfast or lunch. Instead of the usual breakfast foods, try something different, even a potato baked in the microwave and topped with shredded low-fat cheese or vegetarian chili. Don't skip breakfast, even if you are in a hurry.

Here are a few ideas for healthy breakfasts, lunches, or snacks:

• Healthy snacks can include plenty of carrot, celery, broccoli, cauliflower, and low-fat or non-fat yogurt dip.

• Keep plenty of fresh fruit on hand. Make a fruit tray of sliced apples, oranges, bananas, strawberries, pineapple chunks, seedless grapes, and dates or prunes. Dip in low-fat vanilla yogurt.

• Applesauce and graham crackers or peanut butter crackers make a good snack.

• Make frozen fruit bars. You can puree your own fruit or use fruit juice and freeze in bars. This will cut back significantly on the amount of sugar found in store-bought fruit bars.

• Try small strips of thinly sliced ham wrapped around pieces of cubed cantaloupe.

## EASY BROWN BAGS FOR "FIVE A DAY"

❧ Add zucchini, carrot, or sweet pepper strips to your lunch bag.

❧ Try peanut butter and banana sandwiches instead of peanut butter and jam.

❧ Use spinach, tomatoes, and sprouts in sandwiches instead of lettuce.

❧ Marinate a variety of sliced vege-tables with low-fat Italian dressing and use with turkey in a pita pocket.

❧ Add slices of fruit to your sandwich instead of the usual.

❧ Try something different! Go meat-free in sandwiches and make it a veggie sandwich instead.

❧ Include one fresh fruit and one fresh vegetable in all brown bag lunches.

(From the Utah Department of Health Cardiovascular Program. Used by permission.)

• Purchase canned fruits in lite syrup to eat as is, or drain and mix with low-fat plain or vanilla yogurt.

• Thin cheese slices on whole-wheat crackers and a fruit cup, or a fig cookie and milk, make better snacks than candy, pop, and chips.

• Celery with a little peanut butter and a few raisins on top becomes "ants on a log" and is more popular with younger children.

• Whole-wheat mini bagels, whole-wheat pita bread, whole-wheat tortillas, and brown rice crackers are healthy foods to have on hand.

• In separate small plastic bags, put ⅓ cup of a mix of sunflower seeds, peanuts, and almonds for a quick snack on the go. (Don't give to young children. They can choke on nuts.)

• Make a homemade mix of wheat, corn, and oat square cereals with some nuts and bite-sized pretzels mixed in. The store-bought kind has much more salt.

• One cup of air-popped or low-fat microwave popcorn makes a good low calorie snack.

• Melt cheese on whole-wheat tortillas and cut into wedges.

• Let older children make their own "smoothies" with fresh or frozen fruit or fruit juice and skim milk or low-fat yogurt. Add a little vanilla extract for flavoring.

• Spread frozen bananas with peanut butter and slice. Put a toothpick in each slice. The frozen banana can be rolled in crushed nuts or a mixture of oatmeal and brown sugar.

• Make individual pizzas using a whole-wheat English muffin topped with pizza sauce and a slice of cheese toasted under the broiler for a minute or two. (Cheese contains saturated fat and should not be eaten to excess. Low-fat and non-fat cheeses are available.)

• For children, serve salads, potato salads, chicken salads, or almost anything else in an ice cream cone. It will make it more appealing and easier to eat.

• Spread bean dip on a whole-wheat tortilla. (Check labels to find the lowest fat bean dip.)

• Make a fruit punch for an afternoon snack by combining packages of frozen fruits like peaches, raspberries, blueberries, and strawberries with cut up bananas and oranges in a base of pineapple juice, sparkling water, and limeade.

• Turn raw or cooked broccoli into "trees" by cutting broccoli into florettes for the leaves, arranged on a plate with carrots sliced lengthwise to make tree trunks.

• Heat up canned vegetarian chili as a dip for vegetables or with whole-wheat crackers.

• Spread hummus on whole-wheat pita wedges.

• Spoon breakfast cereal into a carton of fruit yogurt.

• An orange, string cheese, and a small bagel make a quick breakfast or snack.

• Add mashed bananas or pieces of dried fruit to pancake or waffle batter.

• Mix up your favorite waffle recipe (preferably using whole wheat) and add cut-up orange or mandarin orange slices to the batter. For a topping, use more sliced oranges mixed with a little orange juice. Or, make whole-wheat pancakes and top with applesauce or fresh berries instead of syrup. Waffles and pancakes are good for dinner too.

• Offer older children a selection of cut-up fruit and wooden skewers to make their own fruit kabobs.

## BROWN BAGGING IT

➤ Pack a low-fat pasta salad or vegetable salad with low-fat dressing.

➤ Pack leftovers from your healthy dinner.

➤ Try tuna packed in water with crackers or bread.

➤ Keep a cup-o-soup on hand.

➤ Keep low-fat frozen entrees in the break room freezer to heat and eat in a rush.

➤ Make sandwiches on bagels, tortillas, English muffins, or pita pockets. Load up with veggies.

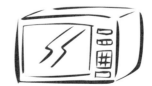

(From the Utah Department of Health Cardiovascular Program. Used by permission.)

• Serve "ladybugs." Core a round red apple and cut in half. Place on a plate with the red side up. Spread small dabs of peanut butter on the apple and put a raisin on each dab.

• For a good on-the-go breakfast or snack, layer cut-up bananas, berries, pineapple tidbits, and vanilla yogurt in a clear plastic drinking cup or parfait glass and top with sliced almonds.

• Shred carrots and add raisins for a quick carrot-raisin salad. Mix with low-fat vanilla yogurt and sprinkle sliced almonds on top if desired.

• Make a breakfast burrito: scramble "Egg Beaters" or similar product, sprinkle with shredded low-fat cheese, and roll up in a warmed tortilla.

• Create a vegetable burrito using a variety of finely chopped vegetables (lettuce, broccoli, cauliflower, green or yellow peppers) with shredded carrots and grated cheese. Roll in a six-inch flour or, better yet, whole-wheat tortilla.

• Make a happy face on a bed of lettuce with hard-boiled egg slices for the eyes, round carrot slices for the mouth, and a radish nose.

• Serve a "rocket salad." Peel a banana and stand it upright in a pineapple ring. Put a maraschino cherry on top of the banana. Decorate the pineapple "rocket base" with shredded carrots for flames.

For more healthy snacks, try the following recipes:

## HOMEMADE SALSA

1 cup fresh diced tomatoes
½ cup corn, fresh or frozen
2 cloves finely diced fresh garlic
½ cup diced onion
1 tablespoon (or less) chopped jalapeno peppers
2 tablespoons lime juice

Combine all of the above ingredients and serve with low-fat baked corn tortilla chips or fresh cut-up veggies.

Calories 33  Cholesterol 0 mg  Protein 1 g  Fiber 1 g  Carbohydrate 8 g  Total fat less than 1 g

(Recipe from Food, Family & Fun, USDA Food and Consumer Service/ Team Nutrition. Used with permission.)

---

## HOMEMADE "CHIPS"

4 corn tortillas (in the dairy section of the supermarket)
Soft butter

Preheat oven to 350° F.

Spread a small amount of softened butter on each tortilla.

Cut tortilla into 8 wedges.

Place wedges in a single layer on a cookie sheet and bake for 10 minutes or until chips are crisp and browned.

(Also try this recipe using flour or whole-wheat tortillas.)

---

## NACHOS

Using the homemade chips from the above recipe, arrange chips on a plate, sprinkle shredded cheese and salsa on top, and microwave in ten-second intervals until cheese is just melted.

---

## PEANUT BUTTER BALLS

¼ cup smooth peanut butter
¼ cup honey
½ cup nonfat dry milk
chopped nuts or coconut

Mix honey and peanut butter; add powdered milk. Roll dough into small balls and roll in nuts or coconut.

---

## BANANA SHAKE FOR TWO

1 cup plain or vanilla yogurt
1 sliced banana
¼ teaspoon vanilla extract
2–4 ice cubes

In a blender, mix yogurt with the sliced banana, vanilla, and ice cubes. As a variation, add ¼ cup chocolate syrup.

## MEXICAN SNACK PIZZAS

whole-wheat English muffins
¼ cup tomato puree
¼ cup canned kidney beans, drained and chopped
1 tablespoon onion, chopped
1 tablespoon green pepper, chopped
½ teaspoon oregano leaves
¼ cup mozzarella cheese (part-skim milk), shredded
¼ cup lettuce, shredded

*Split muffins, toast lightly.*
*Mix tomato puree, beans, onion, green pepper, and oregano and spread on toasted muffin halves. Sprinkle with cheese.*
*Broil until cheese is bubbly (about 2 minutes).*
*Garnish with shredded lettuce.*

## CHILI POPCORN

1 quart popcorn, popped
1 tablespoon margarine, melted
1¼ teaspoons chili powder
¼ teaspoon ground cumin
dash garlic powder

*Mix hot popcorn and margarine.*
*Mix seasonings thoroughly; sprinkle over popcorn. Mix well.*
*Serve immediately.*

## DRIED BANANA OR APPLE CHIPS

Sliced bananas or apples
¼ cup lemon juice

*Peel and thinly slice bananas or apples and dip into lemon juice. Arrange in a single layer on a greased cookie sheet. Bake at 175° F. for two to three hours or until golden. Bake at the longer time if crisper chips are desired. Cool completely before storing.*

## FRUIT JUICE CUBES

1½ tablespoons (1½ envelopes) unflavored gelatin
¾ cup water
6-ounce can frozen grape or apple juice concentrate

*Very lightly grease 9" x 5" inch loaf pan or plastic ice cube trays.*
*Soften gelatin in water in a saucepan for five minutes. Heat over low heat, stirring constantly, until gelatin dissolves. Remove from heat.*
*Add fruit juice concentrate; mix well. Pour into pan.*
*Cover and refrigerate. Chill until set.*
*Cut into 1-inch cubes and serve.*
*Makes about 45 cubes.*

More ideas may be found on the following Web sites:

www.familyfun.com/snackattack (Family Fun magazine)
www.familyfoodzone.com (National Dairy Council)
www.whymilk.com (National Dairy Council)
www.Ilovecheese.com (National Dairy Council)

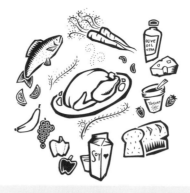

# FUN ACTIVITIES WITH FOOD

- For young children, place a food such as an apple in a paper bag. Let each child take a turn feeling inside the bag and without looking, guess what food is in the bag. Repeat with an orange, tomato, banana, carrots, peanuts, hard cooked egg, and so on.

- Another game for younger children is "What doesn't belong?" Cut out pictures of foods from magazines. Glue them on colored construction paper in groupings depending on the type of food. Add one food that doesn't belong in a group and have children guess which food doesn't belong in that group. For example, a grouping with dairy products could have a picture of a fruit. A grouping of fruits could have a picture of an egg and so forth.

- Also for younger children, make copies of the pictures of fruits and vegetables on pages 192–93 and have children color them. They can then arrange them on construction paper in a rainbow shape. Explain how the reds, oranges, yellows, greens, and blues or violets of the rainbow are also the colors of many of the foods they eat.

- Another good activity for younger children: Make a menu on construction paper, with pictures (or text if the children can read) of healthy foods. Let the children pretend to be waitresses or waiters and present the menu to family members to choose their favorite meals. Cook some of the meals during the coming week.

• Make a word scramble using the names of foods from the pyramid food groups. Use varying degrees of difficulty depending on the ages of the children. For example "LMKI" (MILK) for a younger child and "SSURBESL PURTOSS" (BRUSSELS SPROUTS) for an older child.

• Play "invent a snack." Provide a few healthful ingredients and let everyone invent a snack or sandwich from the foods.

## LESS-FAT DINNER IDEAS

➤ Broil, roast, or stir-fry instead of frying.

➤ Instead of "prime" cuts, choose lower-fat "choice" cuts of meat.

➤ Add frozen veggies to soups, stews, and casseroles.

➤ Remove the skin from poultry.

➤ Limit red meats to no more than a few times a week.

➤ Stir-fry meats in chicken or vegetable broth, water, or pineapple juice.

➤ When using ground meats, cook, drain, and rinse under hot water before proceeding with the recipe.

➤ When making gravy, put ice cubes in meat drippings. Fat will cling to the ice cube for easy removal.

➤ Use lower-fat canned soups and dressings in casseroles.

➤ Cut back or leave the butter or margarine out when preparing most boxed meals.

(From the Utah Department of Health Cardiovascular Program. Used by permission.)

• Play "guess the food." See what happens when someone cannot see or smell their food. Blindfold family members and have them hold their noses (or use a clothespin.) Give them bite-size pieces of different foods and have them guess what they are eating.

• Pay attention to food advertisements on television or in magazines. As a family, go through magazines or watch television and see how many times foods are advertised. (Saturday mornings are a good time to watch for food advertising on TV.) Talk about the types of foods that are being promoted and whether they are nutritious. Discuss the types of nutrients or lack thereof.

• Make up a food. Give it a funny name and try to get your family to "buy" it. Use persuasive techniques they have seen on TV.

• Teach your family the importance of calcium by trying the following experiment. Place a chicken leg bone in a jar with 2 cups water and another chicken leg bone in a jar with 2 cups of vinegar. Put lids on the jars and leave for three or more days. Remove the bones and rinse them. Compare the bones. How flexible is each bone? Bend each bone. The longer the bones are kept in the jars, the better. The vinegar dissolves the calcium, showing that people who do not eat enough foods with calcium have weak, brittle bones.

• Play "Healthy Hopscotch." Draw a hopscotch outline with chalk on the sidewalk and write in the names of the different food groups instead of numbers. Have children throw a beanbag onto the first square. Before each jump they must name a food that belongs in that food group.

• Grow sprouts. You will need alfalfa seeds, plastic zippered sandwich bags, a safety pin, tablespoons, a container for soaking, a dish drainer, pita bread, and grated lowfat cheese.

1. Prepare each bag for sprouting seeds by making tiny holes in the bottom with a safety pin.

2. Make holes in the bottom seam also, so the water will drain well.

3. Put 2 tablespoons of alfalfa seed in each bag (one bag for each family member.)

4. Seal the bags and place them in containers of water to soak overnight.

5. For the next three days, place the bags of seeds in a container of warm water, then drain on a dish drainer for 20 minutes. Store the bags in a cupboard between each soak and drain.

6. After three days, when the seeds have sprouted leaves, place the bags in the light until the leaves turn green.

7. Have family members rinse their sprouts and place them in a piece of pita bread with lowfat grated cheese. Enjoy!

• Talk about healthy options with your family. Explain that family members have choices when it comes to what they eat and how they spend their time. For example, give each person a piece of paper with the following typed on it several times: "I can _____ instead of _____ when _____." A completed sentence might look like this: "I can take a walk instead of watching TV when I get home from school." Go through several options for how they spend their day. Then do the same with food choices. For example: "I could have _____ instead of _____ at _____." Filled out, the sentence could read: "I could have low-fat milk instead of a soft drink at lunch."

• Go on a supermarket "scavenger hunt." For each member of the family, prepare a list of the pyramid food groups and an example of the types of food in each group. Go to the supermarket and give each person a list. Ask them to find at

## QUICK DINNER TIPS FOR "FIVE A DAY"

❥ Use spaghetti squash instead of pasta or rice in your favorite dishes.

❥ Add vegetables to a can of soup.

❥ Substitute finely chopped vegetables with low-fat ricotta cheese for meat in your lasagna recipe.

❥ Cook veggies for 5 minutes in the microwave.

❥ For variety, try a veggie potato bar.

❥ Order extra vegetables when eating out.

❥ Use fruit canned in water or its own juice to top salads.

❥ Garnish your favorite dishes with colorful fruits and vegetables (like tomatoes).

❥ Add pureed or finely minced vegetables to your meatloaf or spaghetti sauce.

❥ For a quick veggie pizza, top a pita pocket with spaghetti sauce, low-fat cheese, and vegetables.

❥ Use greens other than iceberg lettuce in your salads.

❥ Add veggies to your pasta.

❥ Top a baked potato with salsa.

❥ Add more vegetables in casserole recipes.

❥ Use pureed fruit for a sauce over meat.

❥ Add pureed vegetables to thicken sauces, soups, or casseroles.

❥ For a south-of-the-border flavor, make a layered vegetable burrito. Start with rice, beans, cheese, and corn. Then bring on the veggies!

❥ In place of stir-fry or teriyaki sauces, use undiluted frozen 100% juices.

(From the Utah Department of Health Cardiovascular Program. Used by permission.)

least three items from each food group, except the sweets group. If you want, put a time limit on the hunt, say five minutes. When everyone gets back to a designated location in the supermarket, go over everyone's selections and compare nutrition labels. Discuss what meals could be made from the foods that were chosen. Use the ingredients in menus for the upcoming week.

• Play a game that teaches that we eat different parts of plants. Choose items from the following list and have everyone guess what part of the plant it comes from. Then have a tasting party with the foods you have selected. You can do this on several occasions until you have completed the list. When possible, use fresh foods.

*Roots:* beet, onion, carrot, parsnip, potato, radish, rutabaga, sweet potato, turnip

*Stems:* asparagus, bamboo shoots, bok choy, broccoli, celery, rhubarb

*Leaves:* Brussels sprouts, parsley, cabbage, spinach, collards, turnip greens, kale, chard, lettuce, endive, mustard greens, watercress

*Flowers:* broccoli, cauliflower

*Seeds:* lima beans, pinto beans, pumpkin seeds, kidney beans, black beans, sunflower seeds, peas, dry split peas, butter beans, corn

*Fruit:* apple, apricot, artichoke, avocado, grapes, cucumber, banana, pumpkin, squash, bell pepper, date, grapefruit, berries, pear, pineapple, eggplant, plum, tangerine, kiwifruit, mango, melon, orange, papaya, peach, pomegranate, tomato (Source for lists: USDA Team Nutrition)

• Let everyone make an edible artwork. You will need pineapple rings, bananas, tangerines, apples, pears, kiwis, any other fruits you would like, and toothpicks. Drain the pineapple rings and place a ring on a paper plate. Peel the banana and place upright in the center of the pineapple ring. Cut the rest of the fruit into small chunks, wedges, and sections; place them on a plate with a toothpick stuck in each piece. Decorate the banana with the skewered fruit to make a work of edible art.

# A HEALTHY DIET PLAN

A recent article in *Time* magazine stated, "As a society we are clearly in a state of nutritional crisis and in need of radical remedies" (2 September 2002, 49). The article goes on to say "If we were to start from scratch, how would we design a diet to keep our weight under control? For starters, we could concentrate on diets geared for life rather than quick and easy weight loss" (53). The following healthy eating plan is designed to be such a diet.

Calorie counting has gone in and out of favor in the dieting world. Two decades ago it seemed to be all that mattered. Then we were told calories did not count; it was fat grams that mattered. So we all ignored calories and started counting fat grams. The problem with this approach was that we started eating a lot of high-calorie foods, provided the fat content was low. Now we know that calories *do* count, but some calories are more fattening than others. Fatty foods are more easily converted to stored fat than lower-fat foods.

One pound of fat is equal to 3,500 calories. If you eat 500 extra calories per day, you will gain one pound per week. That may sound extreme, but what about 250 extra calories per day, or one pound every two weeks? One extra slice of bread a day could mean an extra ten to twelve pounds a year.

Look over the list of foods you typically eat. If you are having dessert once a day, regularly eating fatty meats like hot

## LOW-FAT BREAKFAST IDEAS

- ❧ Have hot or cold cereal with fat-free milk.
- ❧ Blend up a breakfast shake of low-fat yogurt, 100% juice, and fruit.
- ❧ Make a batch of low-fat muffins and keep them in the freezer. Grab one before heading out the door.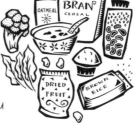
- ❧ Top a bagel with jam or light cream cheese.
- ❧ Carry a low-fat granola bar or breakfast bar to get you going.

(From the Utah Department of Health Cardiovascular Program. Used by permission.)

dogs, ribs, pork chops, and hamburgers, and if you are frequently eating fried foods, salad dressings, cheese, and ice cream, you are due for a change. If your regular snacks are chips, candy, and soda pop you are also due for a change.

Your health is compromised if you are overweight. The National Institute of Health reports that "if you are a woman and your waist measures more than 35 inches, or if you are a man and your waist measures more than 40 inches, you are more likely to develop heart disease, high blood pressure, diabetes, and certain cancers. . . . Overweight people are twice as likely to develop type 2 diabetes (non-insulin-dependent) as people who are not overweight" (*Do You Know the Risks of Being Overweight?* [brochure], Bethesda, Md.: National Institutes of Health, 1998; see also http://137.187.36.5/health/nutri/pubs/health.htm#what, or write to 1 Win Way, Bethesda, MD 20892-3665). Studies show that even losing ten or twenty pounds can improve health. Staying healthy is more than just losing weight or eating right; you also need to exercise and have regular physical checkups.

You need to understand one basic concept that will help you maintain a desirable weight: energy balance. If you eat more calories than your body needs to perform its activities, your body will *store* the calories as fat, and you will gain weight. If you do not eat enough calories to supply your body's needs, or if you exercise and thereby increase your body's energy needs, your body will use stored fat and you will lose weight. In other words, excess calories are used to fuel the exercise instead of being stored as fat. When you have reached your desired weight and you want to maintain

## DARING DESSERTS FOR "FIVE A DAY"

➤ Prepare gelatin with juice instead of water and add fruit slices.

➤ Use pureed canned beans instead of oil (use twice as much as you would oil) in cake mixes for a low-fat treat.

➤ Mash or puree fruit, sweeten lightly, and serve over ice cream.

➤ For a treat, pour lemon-lime soda over cut-up fruit.

➤ Bake pears or bananas with brown sugar and pineapple juice. Stuff them with raisins and spices.

➤ Use canned baby food prunes or applesauce in place of fat in muffins and cake mixes.

➤ Top off a piece of angel food cake with fresh fruit.

(From the Utah Department of Health Cardiovascular Program. Used by permission.)

it, think energy balance. In other words, keep up the exercise and eat sensibly so that you are eating enough to make up for the energy you are expending.

The healthiest and most successful way to weight loss is simple: First, eat less and exercise more. Second, eat primarily vegetables and less red meat. Following these two guidelines in most cases will guarantee successful weight loss without following a specific diet. However some people do best with the structure of a diet. Therefore, a healthy diet is provided below that takes into account the portions and types of food to eat to lose weight.

Not all food, even "good" food, is equally nutritious. Some foods pack more nutrients per calorie than others. To illustrate this concept, the Oregon Dairy Council devised "Pyramid Plus." Pyramid Plus breaks down the USDA's food guide pyramid to show consumers which foods in each group are the healthiest. Four-star foods are the most nutrient-rich and are often the lowest in calories and fat. One-star foods have less nutrition per calorie. They are not "bad" foods, just foods to choose less often. (Most of the foods in the vegetable and fruit groups are still low in calories and low in fat, regardless of their rating.) The charts on the following pages summarize the Oregon Dairy Council's Pyramid Plus. Nutrients are listed under each food group heading (*Pyramid Plus: A Star-Studded Guide to Food Choices for Better Health* [brochure], Nutrition Education Services/Oregon Dairy Council, 1997. For more information about Pyramid Plus, call 503-229-5033).

The number of calories you can eat to lose weight is highly individual. It will vary according to age, sex, height, level of activity, and heredity. Pregnant or nursing women, older adults, teenagers, children, athletes, and men each have different food needs. Most children, teenage girls, *active* women,

# Breads & Cereals

### Supplies: Fiber, complex carbohydrates, thiamin, iron, niacin

| ★★★★ (Most Nutrients) | ★★★ | ★★ | ★ (Fewest Nutrients) |
|---|---|---|---|
| Barley | Brown rice | Flour tortillas | Cornbread |
| Bulgur | Bran muffin | Bagel | Fruit or nut bread |
| Bran or whole-grain cereals | Whole-grain crackers | Enriched breads | Biscuit |
| Popcorn (air-popped or light microwave) | Soft pretzel | Enriched rice | Stuffing |
| Whole-grain breads | English muffin | Pancakes | Croissant |
| Oatmeal | Enriched pasta | Waffles | |
| Whole-grain pasta | Popcorn (oil-popped) | Graham crackers | |
| Corn or whole-wheat tortillas | | Saltines | |
| | | Sweetened cereal | |
| | | Dry pretzels | |

# Vegetables

### Supplies: Folic acid, vitamins A and C, fiber

| ★★★★ (Most Nutrients) | ★★★ | ★★ | ★ (Fewest Nutrients) |
|---|---|---|---|
| Red and green bell peppers | Cabbage | Beets | Eggplant |
| Mustard greens | Chard | Cucumber | Corn |
| Bok choy | Asparagus | Celery | Avocado |
| Spinach | Kale | Jicama | Potato |
| Leaf lettuce | Vegetable juice | Artichoke | |
| Broccoli | Brussels sprouts | Peas | |
| Carrots | Salsa | Mushrooms | |
| Cauliflower | Iceberg lettuce | | |
| | Sweet potato | | |
| | Tomato | | |
| | Snow peas | | |
| | Zucchini | | |
| | Okra | | |
| | Winter squash | | |
| | Green beans | | |

# Fruits

## Supplies: Folic acid, vitamins A and C, fiber

| ★★★★ (Most Nutrients) | ★★★ | ★★ | ★ (Fewest Nutrients) |
|---|---|---|---|
| Papaya | Honeydew | Peach | Pear |
| Strawberries | Raspberries | Nectarine | Apple |
| Kiwi | Apricots | Banana | Dried fruit |
| Orange | Rhubarb | Plum | Grapes |
| Grapefruit | Pineapple | Cherries | Raisins |
| Cantaloupe | Watermelon | Frozen fruit | |
| Mandarin oranges | Blueberries | juice bar | |
| Mango | | Canned fruit | |

# Milk & Milk Products

## Supplies: Calcium, riboflavin, protein

| ★★★★ (Most Nutrients) | ★★★ | ★★ | ★ (Fewest Nutrients) |
|---|---|---|---|
| Nonfat plain yogurt | Part-skim ricotta cheese | Custard | Cottage cheese |
| Nonfat milk | Whole milk | Low-fat frozen yogurt | Ice cream |
| Nonfat cream cheese | Regular-fat cheese | Light ice cream | Nonfat sour cream |
| Nonfat fruit yogurt | Low-fat chocolate milk (1%) | Milkshake | |
| Low-fat milk (1%) | Low-fat fruit yogurt | | |
| Buttermilk | Nonfat frozen yogurt | | |
| Low-fat cheese | Pudding | | |
| Reduced-fat milk (2%) | | | |

# Meat & Meat Alternatives

## Supplies: Iron, protein, niacin, thiamin, zinc, vitamin B12

| ★★★★ (Most Nutrients) | ★★★ | ★★ | ★ (Fewest Nutrients) |
|---|---|---|---|
| Fish | Beef (rib, chuck, flank, and ground) | Hot dogs | Peanut butter |
| Shellfish | Egg substitute | Pork sausage | Bologna |
| Poultry (light meat, skinless) | Ham (lean) | Chicken nuggets | |
| Turkey ham | Tofu | Fish sticks | |
| Beef (round and sirloin) | Veal and lamb (leg and loin) | Nuts and seeds | |
| Pork (tenderloin) | Poultry (dark meat with skin) | | |
| Veal (leg and shoulder) | Pork (loin chop and rib) | | |
| Lentils | Canadian bacon | | |
| | Poultry sausage | | |
| | Dried beans and peas | | |
| | Eggs | | |

*Source: Nutrition Education Services/Oregon Dairy Council.*

and sedentary men need to eat more than the minimum but less than the maximum number of servings recommended for each food group. Active men, very active women, and teenage boys can usually consume the maximum number of servings recommended on the pyramid. (If you are pregnant or nursing, ask your doctor about your dietary needs.)

Serving sizes on nutrition facts labels are based on a 2,000-calorie diet. The 2,000-calorie diet is based on what a "typical" person eats who is not trying to lose weight. Eating 2,000 calories a day, even at the maintenance phase of this diet, may be too high for those who are older or not particularly active.

If you want to lose weight, do the following, and remember that calorie levels are approximate. For family members that are tall or very active, begin at a higher calorie range. Women should not eat fewer than 1,200 calories a day, but may, in time, be able to maintain a desirable weight while eating more than 1,800 calories a day.

1. Start off at the lower calorie range: 1,200 to 1,400 calories is a good place for most women to begin if they want to lose weight and are of average height (5' 4") and activity. Start by eating the minimum number of servings suggested per day for each food group *and* choosing foods primarily from the four-star list provided by the Oregon Dairy Council. If you lose more than two pounds per week, add another serving of a four-star food from one of the groups. Likewise, do not eat fewer than the minimum number of servings recommended per day, even if you do not see immediate results. You will soon. The minimum number of servings was calculated to give you just the right amounts of vitamins, minerals, carbohydrates, and protein your body needs.

2. When you have made significant progress, you can try going up to a mid-calorie range (between 1,400 and 1,600 calories a day for average women). To do this, stick with eating the minimum number of servings, but add to your food choices by selecting from the three-star listings as well as the four. Monitor how you are doing. You can add or subtract the number of servings and change the nutrient categories accordingly. Your activity level should be increasing as well, so keep exercising.

3. When you have reached your desired weight, or even before, depending on your level of activity, your age, and your unique body, start eating in the maintenance range (between 1,600 and 1,800 calories a day for an average woman). This

means you will still be eating the minimum number of servings each day, but the range of foods to choose from can now
include those in the two-star category. It is easy to adjust your
choices if necessary. You may decide to choose two-star foods
only occasionally, and instead eat more servings from the
fruit, vegetable, and bread groups. (Remember to eat mostly
whole grains.) You will still need to eat the minimum number of servings from each group. Don't cut out one serving of
milk in order to eat more fruits, vegetables, and bread.
Because most of the vegetables are so low in calories and fat,
you should be able to eat more servings from this food group
anyway. *The more you exercise, the more liberal you can be in
your choices.*

*This is very important*: Eat the maximum calories you can
while still losing weight. In other words, if you are losing 1½
to 2 pounds a week on 1,400 calories per day, don't drop to
1,200 calories. If you take this approach, you will be more
likely to stick with your diet and you will have more energy.

If you do not need to lose weight, but just want to have a
healthier diet, choose foods from the four-star and three-star
categories, keeping desserts and fatty foods to a minimum.
Keep exercising.

Following are breakfast, lunch, dinner, and snack ideas for
the low-calorie plan. The low-calorie plan (1,200–1,400 calories per day) works best for women over thirty. Younger family members, or those who need to lose less than ten pounds,
can get by with eating more calories and exercising a bit
more. Make up your own menus as well. Recipes for the
starred items are included in the "More Recipes" chapter.

# Breakfast

1 cup mixed fruit—kiwi, strawberries, and mandarin
    oranges (2 fruits)

½ cup plain yogurt (½ milk)—try flavoring the yogurt with a
little vanilla or cinnamon
1 slice whole-wheat toast with a little butter or margarine
(1 bread)

---

1 egg, fried, using vegetable spray (½ meat)
1 slice whole-wheat toast with a little butter or margarine
(l bread)
½ grapefruit (1 fruit)

---

1 cup cooked whole-grain cereal (2 breads)
1 cup skim milk (1 milk)
6 ounces orange juice (1 fruit)

---

1 whole-grain bagel with a little butter or margarine
(2 breads)
1 cup fruit smoothie* (1 fruit, 1 milk)

---

1 cup shredded wheat with small banana (2 breads, 1 fruit),
or any cold cereal with ½ cup sliced fruit
½ cup skim milk (½ milk)
1 slice toast with a little butter or margarine (1 bread)

---

2 fruit bran muffins* (2 breads, 1 fruit)
1 cup skim milk (1 milk)

---

½ toasted whole-wheat English muffin with 1 slice tomato
and 1 thin slice low-fat cheese, broiled (1 bread, ½ milk)
½ grapefruit (1 fruit)
½ cup skim milk (½ milk)

---

1 cup homemade granola* (2 breads, ½ meat, 1 fruit)
1 cup skim milk (1 milk)

2 eggs, scrambled, using one yolk and two whites (1 meat)
1 piece whole-wheat toast with 1 tablespoon jam (1 bread,
   ½ fruit)
½ cup strawberries (1 fruit)
1 cup skim milk (1 milk)

1 whole-wheat tortilla with 1 scrambled egg and 1 tablespoon
   salsa (1 bread, ½ meat)
6 ounces fruit juice (1 fruit)

1 two-egg omelet with mushrooms, onions, peppers,
   sprouts, and tomatoes (1 meat, 1 vegetable)
½ whole-grain English muffin with a little butter or
   margarine (1 bread)
1 orange (1 fruit)

## Lunch

You can take many of these to work or school, or eat
equivalents if you are going out to lunch. Have with ice water
and a slice of lemon.

½ can tuna (1 meat)
1 cup chopped tomato and celery (1 vegetable)
1 cup lettuce or spinach (1 vegetable )
1 whole-wheat roll (1 bread)
1 cup plain nonfat yogurt (1 milk)

1 corn tortilla, cooked a few seconds on each side in pan
   sprayed with vegetable oil (1 bread) filled with:
½ can vegetarian no-fat chili or other bean (1 meat)
Chopped lettuce and tomatoes (1 vegetable)
1½ ounces grated nonfat cheese (1 milk)

1½ cups white bean soup* (1 vegetable, 1 meat)
1 whole-wheat roll (1 bread)
1 cup lettuce or spinach with 1 tablespoon low-calorie
   dressing (1 vegetable)

---

½ whole-wheat pita (1 bread) filled with:
2 ounces chopped chicken mixed with 1 teaspoon low-fat
   mayo (1 meat)
chopped onion, tomato, and celery (1 vegetable)

---

2 slices whole-wheat bread (2 breads) topped and broiled
   with:
cucumber and tomato slices (1 vegetable)
1½ ounces low-fat cheese, sliced thin (1 milk)

---

½ whole-grain English muffin (1 bread) topped and broiled
   with:
2 ounces thin-sliced turkey ham (1 meat)
1 thin slice low-fat cheese (½ milk)
1 tomato, sliced (1 vegetable)

---

1½ cups minestrone soup* (1 meat, 1 vegetable)
1 whole-wheat roll with a little butter or margarine
   (1 bread)
1 cup lettuce or spinach with 1 tablespoon low-fat, low-
   calorie dressing (1 vegetable)

---

Egg-salad sandwich with 1 egg and 1 teaspoon low-fat mayo
   (½ meat)
2 slices whole-grain bread (2 breads)
1 cup cooked green beans with a little butter or margarine
   (2 vegetables)

1 cup carrot-raisin salad* (1 vegetable, 1 fruit, ½ milk)
4 small, plain whole-grain crackers (1 bread)
1 cup vegetable soup* (1 vegetable)

Tuna salad with ½ can tuna, 1 tablespoon low-fat mayon-
    naise, and chopped cucumbers (1 meat, ½ vegetable)
2 slices whole-grain bread (2 breads)
1 cantaloupe section, approximately ¼ of the fruit (1 fruit)

Vegetable quesadillas* (2 bread, 1 milk, 1 vegetable)
1 hard-boiled egg (½ meat)
½ mango or papaya (1 fruit)

1 tomato, stuffed with 3 ounces canned salmon, mixed with
    1 tablespoon low-fat mayonnaise (1 vegetable, 1 meat)
½ whole-wheat roll (1 bread)

1 cup lettuce and spinach salad with 1 tablespoon low-fat
    dressing (1 vegetable)
1 small baked potato (1 vegetable) topped with:
1 cup vegetarian low-fat chili or refried beans (½ meat)
1½ ounces low-fat cheese (1 milk)

½ cup kiwi and strawberries (1 fruit)
1 small baked potato (1 vegetable) topped with:
½ cup cooked broccoli (1 vegetable)
1½ ounces low-fat cheese (1 milk)

1 cup whole-wheat pasta or regular pasta (2 breads)
½ cup homemade pasta sauce* (½ vegetable)
1 cup cooked broccoli (2 vegetables)

3 ounces lean roast beef, turkey, or chicken (1 meat) on
2 slices rye or whole-wheat bread (2 breads)
2 tablespoons low-fat mayonnaise
1 cup lettuce with 1 chopped tomato, celery, sprouts
 (2 vegetables)

## Dinner

Have these meals with water or milk, depending on the
number of milk servings you have already had for the day. If
you didn't have a leafy salad for lunch, have one for dinner.
Try not to have meat for dinner if you had meat for lunch
(this does not include fish, which can be eaten more often
because it is lower in fat, calories, and cholesterol than other
meats). Choose a meat substitute instead. Some days try to
have meat substitutes for both lunch and dinner. For
example, have an omelet for lunch and a vegetable or bean
soup for dinner. Check the number of servings you've had so
far in the day.

Tuna pasta salad* (1 meat, 1 fruit, 2 breads)
1 cup cooked carrots or broccoli (2 vegetables)

Turkey casserole* with broccoli and brown rice (1 meat,
 1 vegetable, 2 breads)
1 cup roasted green and red peppers (2 vegetables)

1 cup whole-grain or ½ whole grain and ½ regular spaghetti
 with homemade pasta sauce* (2 breads, 2 vegetables)
1 cup steamed green beans with oregano (2 vegetables)

1 small sweet potato with a little butter and ½ teaspoon
 brown sugar, if desired (1 vegetable)

1 cup broccoli (2 vegetables)
3 ounces any type baked fish, with low-fat sauce (1 meat)
1 whole-wheat roll (1 bread)

---

Stuffed baked potato (1 vegetable) with:
1½ ounces cheese (1 milk)
½ cup broccoli or ½ cup vegetarian low-fat chili (1 vegetable
    or 1 meat)

---

Fish stew* (1 or 2 meats, 1 or 2 vegetables)
1 whole-grain roll (1 bread)
Lettuce and spinach salad with low-fat, low-calorie dressing
    (1 vegetable)

---

Oriental pork tenderloin with teriyaki or sweet and sour
    sauce, pineapple, and green peppers (1 meat, 1 fruit,
    1 vegetable)
1 cup brown rice or mixed brown and white rice (2 breads)

---

Italian chicken* (1 meat, 1 vegetable)
1 small baked potato (1 vegetable)
1 cup lightly buttered green beans (1 vegetable)

---

Curry chicken* (1 meat)
½ or 1 cup wild rice (1 or 2 breads)
½ cup peas (1 vegetable)

---

Bagel pizza* (2 breads, 1 milk, 1 vegetable)
Lettuce and spinach salad with low-fat, low-calorie dressing
    (1 vegetable)

---

2 tortillas with 1/2 cup black beans and salsa (2 breads,
    1 meat)

½ cup cooked corn, lightly buttered (1 vegetable)
1 orange (1 fruit)

---

2-egg omelet with vegetables (1 meat, 1 vegetable)
1 roasted potato (1 vegetable)

---

Fish parmesan* (1 meat, 1 milk)
½ cup wild or brown rice (1 bread)
½ cup cooked carrots (1 vegetable)

---

Chicken dijon* (1 meat)
½ cup whole-wheat pasta with a little butter (1 bread)
½ cup cooked green beans (1 vegetable)

---

Bean and rice casserole (1 meat, 1 bread)
Green salad with low-calorie, low-fat dressing (1 vegetable)
Cold vegetable plate with plain yogurt dip (1 or 2 vegetables,
    1 milk)

## Snacks

Snacks are optional, but you may eat one to three per day.
Don't forget, however, that they contribute to your overall
daily consumption from each food group.

---

Vegetable platter of carrots, snow peas, cauliflower, and
    broccoli (1 or 2 vegetables). This can be served with non-
    fat plain yogurt for a dip (½ milk).

---

Fruit, especially those with four stars (1 fruit)

---

1 cup plain, air-popped popcorn. If you buy the packaged
    microwave kind, make sure there is no fat (3 cups
    plain = 1 bread).

---

½ whole-grain English muffin (1 bread)

---

½ cup plain, low-fat yogurt with 3 or 4 whole-grain crackers (½ milk, 1 bread)

If you are following the mid-calorie plan, use fruits and vegetables from all the categories in Pyramid Plus and try three-starred items from the other food groups. When you are eating at the maintenance level, choose from the two-star range occasionally. Your menus can now include: a wider selection of meat; more white potatoes; whole-grain pancakes or waffles for any meal; pita bread; baked corn tortilla chips with salsa for a snack; or graham crackers. Snacks can also include ⅓ cup nuts as well as frozen fruit-juice bars. Instead of choosing some of the higher-calorie foods, you may choose to eat more or larger servings of the low-calorie foods. Monitor your progress and be aware of the number of servings and serving sizes you eat each day.

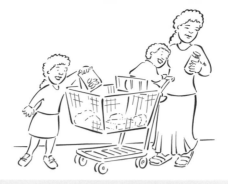

# BUYING AND PREPARING FOOD

## Shopping for Food

Here are some suggestions for your next grocery shopping trip that will help in selecting healthier foods. If you always have the basic items listed below on hand, it will be easy to put together a quick meal.

• Cut down on red meat purchases. This alone will reduce your food bill. Buy lean cuts. Often the meat department will trim the remaining visible fat for you. Ask the butcher's advice for the leanest cuts of meat. These would include pork tenderloin, round tip roast, and sirloin. Buy more fish than you are accustomed to. Have cans of **tuna, salmon,** and **clams** on hand. Add them to pasta or beans for a quick meal. Thinner cuts of meat cook the fastest. The white meat of poultry is lower in fat. Buy skinned chicken breast, or skin the chicken before you cook it.

• Look for low-fat dairy products, such as skim or one-percent milk, low-fat or nonfat yogurt, and low-fat cheeses. Have **powdered nonfat milk** on hand.

• Buy cooking oils that are unsaturated or monounsaturated, such as canola oil, corn oil, olive oil, and soybean oil.

• Select breads, bagels, and English muffins made from whole-wheat, rye, bran, or corn flour or corn meal. Read the nutrition facts label on the bread. Some "wheat" bread has

150

no more fiber than white bread. Even if the bread says "multigrain," check the label. "Whole wheat" or "whole grain" means the food contains a bran layer, which is the outer coating of the grain and is high in fiber.

• Buy whole-wheat flour, but keep it in the refrigerator or freezer, because its shelf life is shorter than white flour. Try **whole-wheat pancake mixes** and **whole-grain** or **bran cereals, whole-wheat pasta, brown rice,** and **bulgur wheat**. You do not need to switch entirely to whole grains. And definitely do not try to do so all at once—the body needs time to get used to digesting whole grains. Products made with white flour are not "bad." Because they are fortified they are still nutritious, but they lack the fiber of whole-grain products and are converted into sugar by the body more rapidly. Try mixing **brown** and **white rice,** or **whole-grain** and regular **pasta**. Cook up several batches of brown rice and freeze to save time. Do not be fooled by colored pastas. Vegetable extracts are used to add color, but that is about all that is added. It is still regular pasta.

• **Dry beans** are inexpensive and good to have on hand, but except for split peas and lentils, they have to be soaked several hours or overnight. So also have plenty of **canned beans** like **cannellini, kidney, black, garbanzo,** and **pinto** to mix with pastas, greens, and vegetables for fast hot or cold meals. Rinse canned beans to remove the salt. Try **vegetarian refried beans, chili,** and **baked beans**. Use them as toppings on potatoes if you do not want to eat them plain. As little as one-half cup of beans is a good addition to daily protein requirements.

• Keep **honey, balsamic vinegar,** and **dijon mustard** in your pantry to use for coating fish and chicken.

• **Canned fat-free evaporated milk** can be mixed with dijon mustard to make a creamy sauce for meats.

• Have on hand **low-sodium soy, Worcestershire,** and **teriyaki sauces, blackening seasoning,** bottled or packaged **pesto sauce, orange marmalade, peach preserves, apricot preserves, cranberry sauce,** and **currant jelly** for glazing meats and fish.

• Reduced-sodium, fat-free **chicken** and **beef broth, reduced-sodium canned chopped tomatoes, salsa, frozen stir-fry vegetables,** and **minced garlic** are good for last-minute meals.

• You will also need **olive** and **sesame oils** and the following seasonings: **garlic-pepper, lemon-herb,** and **Mexican seasonings. Key lime juice** is a good staple as well.

• **Cornflake crumbs** and **plain** or **Italian-seasoned bread crumbs** are good to have for coating chicken and fish for baking to get a crunchy crust without frying.

• Stock up on **grains, pastas,** and **rice,** especially **whole wheat.** Buy **orzo** and **couscous,** which cook up quickly. With some fresh produce, beans, and grains, several last-minute, healthy dinners can be prepared.

• **Taco shells** and **tortillas,** especially the whole-wheat kind, are good sources of complex carbohydrates. Avoid pre-made taco shells—they are deep-fat fried. Buy them uncooked and fry your own by spraying a pan with a little vegetable spray and cooking on both sides for two minutes or less, then folding. Have **whole-wheat pita bread** on hand as well.

• Keep fresh **fruits** and **vegetables** available for your family. **Romaine lettuce** has six times the vitamin C and eight times the beta-carotene as iceberg lettuce. This does not mean iceberg lettuce is "bad," but it demonstrates the need to pick a variety of produce. Have fresh **spinach** on hand as well as **salad greens, red and green peppers, lemons, tomatoes,** and **zucchini**. When possible, buy produce when the foods are in season and eat them right away. Any time the fruit or vegetable is processed, some of the nutrients are lost. However, fresh food kept in the refrigerator for days looses a substantial amount of nutrients. Often canned or frozen vegetables are actually "fresher" because the time lapse from picked to processed is short. If you like to garden and have the space, the best solution is to grow as much as you can and eat it immediately or process it immediately.

• **Canned** and **dried fruit** are good too, but they contain more sugar. Peaches in light syrup have two teaspoons of added sugar per half-cup serving; heavy syrup has four teaspoons of added sugar. Look for fruits packed in their own juices. **Frozen berries** are good to have on hand and they often are prepared without sugar.

• When you buy **canned vegetables**, get the no-salt or low-salt canned kind; all others can be rinsed. To get used to more variety, buy some vegetables you would not ordinarily choose.

## Preparing Food

When it comes time to prepare the foods, there are choices that will result in healthier meals.

• Serve raw vegetables such as carrots, broccoli, cauliflower, and snow peas more often, but don't leave them sitting in the refrigerator for several days. Raw vegetables contain natural enzymes and phytonutrients that are depleted during the cooking process.

• Steam vegetables—less nutrients are lost this way. Also, the liquid used to cook vegetables contains some dissolved vitamins and can be used in other dishes. In general, the shorter the cooking time, the more nutrients are preserved. High heat also destroys vitamins.

## PREPARING BAKED GOODS WITH LESS FAT

- ◆ Use two egg whites in place of one whole egg in most quick breads, cookies, and cakes.
- ◆ Cut most fat in recipes by ⅓ to ½ safely. Replace with another ingredient, such as pureed prunes, carrots, or bananas.
- ◆ When using mixes, replace most or all the fat with applesauce, buttermilk, or yogurt.
- ◆ Use three tablespoons of cocoa in place of each ounce of unsweetened baking chocolate.
- ◆ Cut back on nuts, chocolate chips, and other high-fat mix-ins. Toast nuts before adding to increase flavor, and use mini-chips to spread out the chocolate flavor more.
- ◆ Add a small amount of vanilla, cinnamon, or nutmeg to enhance flavor when fat and sugar are reduced.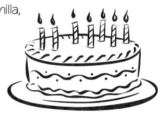
- ◆ Use phyllo dough in place of a pie crust.

(From the Utah Department of Health Cardiovascular Program. Used by permission.)

• Bake, steam, boil, microwave, or broil food instead of frying it. A fried pork chop has 16 grams of fat, while a lean piece of roast pork has half that amount. A three-ounce piece of fried chicken has 12 grams of fat, compared to a piece of baked chicken with 8 fat grams.

• Trim off the fat from meats, and skin poultry and fish. Cook poultry on a rack to keep it out of the drippings.

• Skim fat from soups and gravies. After the soups or gravies are refrigerated it is easier to remove much of the fat.

- Cook with skim milk. To save money, use powdered non-fat milk. Mix two quarts and keep in the refrigerator for cooking.
  - Use low-fat, low-calorie mayonnaise and salad dressings.
  - Use low-fat yogurt instead of sour cream.
  - Sauté or stir-fry and use less fat.
  - To cut cholesterol, substitute one whole egg and one egg white in recipes that call for two whole eggs.
  - Make homemade soups and freeze enough for meals later. Included in the recipe section is a way to thicken soups without using much fat.
  - Use one-third less oil than the recipe calls for when baking. Experiment to see what works best. Pureed fruit can be used in place of some of the fat in recipes. The fruit adds moisture, but because it does not melt like fat, the outcome is changed somewhat. Replace about one-fourth to one-half of the fat in recipes and test the quality. It may be necessary to maintain at least one tablespoon of fat per cup of flour in the recipe. Longer baking time may be needed because the fruit will make the recipe extra moist.
  - Substitute whole grain flour for part of the all-purpose flour called for in recipes.
  - Reduce salt by one-half of the amount called for in a recipe.
  - Mash kidney beans or pinto beans and use in tacos or burritos in place of half of the ground beef.
  - Invest in a slow-cooker (better known as a Crock-pot) to prepare nutritious meals that can be cooking while you are busy.

# Shopping List

apricot preserves
baked beans
balsamic vinegar
beans, dry
beef broth
blackening seasoning
bran cereals
bread crumbs (plain or Italian-
   seasoned)
brown rice
bulgur wheat
canned beans (cannellini, kidney, black, garbanzo, pinto)
canned chopped tomatoes
canned fat-free evaporated milk
canned fruit
canned vegetables
chicken
chicken broth
chili
cornflake crumbs
couscous
cranberry sauce
currant jelly
dijon mustard
dried fruit
frozen berries
frozen stir-fry vegetables
fruits
garlic-pepper seasoning
grains
honey
Key lime juice
lemon-herb seasoning

lemons
Mexican seasoning
minced garlic
olive oil
orange marmalade
orzo
pastas
peach preserves
pesto sauce
powdered nonfat milk
red and green peppers
reduced-sodium canned
   chopped tomatoes
romaine lettuce
salad greens
salsa
sesame oil
soy sauce, low-sodium
spinach
taco shells
teriyaki sauce, low sodium
tomatoes
tortillas
vegetables
vegetarian refried beans
white rice
whole-grain cereals
whole-wheat pancake mixes
whole-wheat pasta
whole-wheat pita bread
Worcestershire sauce, low
   sodium
zucchini

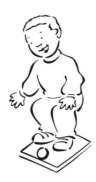

# IF YOUR CHILD IS OVERWEIGHT

The Weight Control Information Network (www.niddk. nih.gov) has published information sheets to help parents who have overweight children. The following ideas are adapted from one of these called "Helping Your Overweight Child."

A child's diet and activity level play a large part in determining whether he or she is overweight. Fast food, soda pop, chips, and candy, combined with hours of television, computer, and video games have contributed to a potential health crisis for today's children.

Children's health experts suggest:

• Support, accept, and encourage your children. They need to know you love them whatever their weight. At the same time, talk with them and let them share their feelings. Let them know you are there to help them.

• Involve the family in changing the family's lifestyle.

• Increase the family's physical activity by:

1. Becoming more active yourself.
2. Planning exercise activities in which everyone can participate.
3. Being sensitive if your overweight child is embarrassed or finds the activity too difficult.
4. Cutting back on the amount of time the family spends in watching TV and other sedentary activities.

5. Teaching and practicing healthy eating habits. Learn more about nutrition and give your children healthy meal options.

• Do not place your child on a restrictive diet unless a doctor supervises one for medical reasons. Only limit sweets, fast food, soda pop, and so on. Offer your child a variety of fruits, vegetables, and whole grains.

• Guide your family's choices rather than dictate foods. If you make a variety of healthy foods available in the house, you will help your children learn how to make wise choices.

• Encourage your children to eat slowly.

• Eat meals together as a family

• Reduce the amount of saturated fat in your family's diet. If you have children under two years old, they should still be drinking whole milk.

• Do not overly restrict treats. Teach your children moderation.

• Involve children in food shopping and preparing meals.

• Plan nutritious snacks.

• Do not use food to punish or reward.

• Discourage eating or snacking in front of the TV. Overeating is more likely to occur if children are paying attention to the TV instead of what and how much they are eating.

• Set a good example.

• Make sure meals outside the home are balanced, whether at school or at restaurants.

• Seek help if necessary. The Weight Control Information Network (WIN) has a list of university-based medical centers. Contact WIN at 202-828-1025, fax 202-828-1028, or e-mail at win@info.niddk.nih.gov. You can also call the National Center for Nutrition and Dietetics of the American Dietetic Association at 800-366-1655 to get the name of a registered dietician in your area. Also available from the Cooperative

Extension, University of California, Division of Agriculture and Natural Resources is a pamphlet called "If My Child Is Too Fat, What Should I Do About It?" by J. Ikeda. Call 415-642-2431 and ask for publication #21455.

• Look for a weight-control program with the following characteristics:

1. It is staffed with a variety of health professionals, including registered dieticians, exercise physiologists, pediatricians or family physicians, and psychiatrists or psychologists.
2. It performs a medical evaluation of your child. Weight, growth, and health should be reviewed and monitored by health professionals on a regular basis.
3. Its programs are adapted to the specific age and capability of your child.
4. It focuses on behavioral changes.
5. It teaches your child how to select a variety of foods in appropriate portions.
6. It encourages daily activity and limits sedentary activity, like watching TV.
7. It focuses on the whole family, not just the overweight child.
8. It includes a maintenance program and support and referral resources to reinforce new behaviors and deal with underlying issues that contributed to the child being overweight.

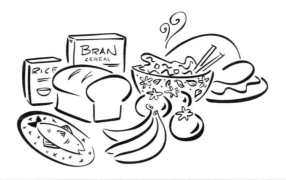

# MORE RECIPES

## Fruits and Vegetables

Recipes with a * are included in the healthy diet plan meals on pages 141–49.

### HERBED VEGETABLE COMBO

These steamed vegetables with herb seasonings add color and flavor to a meal without adding fat or salt.

2 tablespoons water
1 cup zucchini squash, thinly sliced
1¼ cups yellow squash, thinly sliced
½ cup green pepper, cut into 2-inch strips
¼ cup celery, cut into 2-inch strips
¼ cup onion, chopped
½ teaspoon caraway seed
⅛ teaspoon garlic powder
1 medium tomato, cut into 8 wedges

*Heat water in a large frying pan. Add squash, green pepper, celery, and onion. Cover and cook over moderate heat until the vegetables are tender-crisp—about 4 minutes. Sprinkle seasonings over vegetables. Top with tomato wedges. Cover and cook over low heat until tomato wedges are just heated—about 2 minutes. Makes 4 ¾-cup servings*

*Nutrients:*

*25 calories, trace total fat, trace saturated fatty acids, 0 mg cholesterol, 10 mg sodium.*

*Source: United States Department of Agriculture.*

## BAKED APPLES

4 medium cooking apples
4 tablespoons raisins
¾ cup water
½ teaspoon cinnamon

*Preheat oven to 350° F. Remove cores from apples, leaving ½ inch of the core at bottom of the apple. Peel top one-third of apple. Arrange apples in baking pan. Put 1 tablespoon of raisins in the center of each apple. Pour water over apples. Sprinkle cinnamon over apples. Bake 45 to 60 minutes or until tender. Spoon liquid from pan over apples one or two times during baking. Makes 4 servings; 1 apple each.*

*Nutrients:*

*150 calories, 1 g total fat, 0 mg cholesterol, 0 mg sodium.*

*Source: United States Department of Agriculture.*

---

## FRUIT SMOOTHIE*

1½ cups skim or 1 percent milk
6-ounce can frozen orange or other juice (softened)
1 cup water
1½ teaspoons vanilla extract

*Pour milk in large bowl or blender. Add other ingredients and whisk or blend until foamy. Serve immediately.*

*Source: University of Illinois at Urbana-Champaign.*

# Salads

## CARROT-RAISIN SALAD*

2 cups shredded carrots
¹/₂ cup raisins
2 tablespoons fat-free mayonnaise
¹/₄ cup plain, nonfat yogurt
2 tablespoons lemon juice

*Shred carrots and combine with other ingredients; chill. Makes 6 servings.*

*Nutrients:*

*74 calories, 21% DV total fat, 2 mg cholesterol, 56 mg sodium, 74% DV carbohydrate, 5% DV protein, 33 mg calcium, 0.5 mg iron.*

*Source: University of Utah Nutrition Clinic.*

## PASTA SALAD

¾ cup elbow macaroni, uncooked
10-ounce package frozen mixed vegetables
⅓ medium green pepper, chopped
2 tablespoons onion, chopped
¼ cup low-fat Italian dressing

*Cook macaroni and frozen vegetables according to package directions. Leave out the salt. Drain. Add the green pepper, onion, and low-fat Italian dressing. Mix all ingredients. Chill well. Makes 4 1-cup servings.*

*Nutrients:*

*135 calories, 2 g total fat, 0 mg cholesterol, 145 mg sodium.*

*Source: United States Department of Agriculture.*

## CRUNCHY PEA SALAD

1½ cups USA split peas, rinsed
3 cups water
1½ cups instant rice, cooked
8-ounce can water chestnuts, diced
3 bunches green onions, chopped
½ cup chopped celery

Dressing:
1 cup cholesterol-free mayonnaise
½ cup chili sauce
Few drops Tabasco sauce
1 tablespoon horseradish (optional)
¼ cup sweet red pepper sauce (optional)

*Cook the split peas in boiling water for 25 to 30 minutes. Peas should be tender, not mushy. Drain, rinse, and chill. Chill cooked rice. Combine the peas and rice with the water chestnuts, green onions, and celery. Serve with dressing.*

*For dressing combine mayonnaise, chili sauce, Tabasco sauce, horseradish, and pepper sauce. Serves 12.*

*Nutrients:*

*256 calories, 9 g total fat, 0 mg cholesterol, 206 mg sodium, 38 g carbohydrate, 1 g dietary fiber, 6 g protein.*

*Source: USA Dry Pea and Lentil Council, Moscow, Idaho.*

## LENTIL CONFETTI SALAD

3 cups water
1 cup USA lentils, rinsed
1 cup rice, cooked and warm
1 large tomato, seeded and diced
1 tablespoon parsley, chopped
½ cup onion, chopped
½ cup celery, chopped
¼ cup pimento-stuffed olives, sliced
¼ cup sweet green pepper, diced
½ cup light Italian dressing

Garnish:

cucumbers and red onion rings, sliced

*In a saucepan, pour water over lentils, bring to a boil, and simmer 20 minutes or until lentils are tender. Combine drained lentils with rice and all vegetables. Toss lightly with dressing. Place on a ring of cucumbers and garnish with red onion rings. Serves 8.*

*Nutrients:*

*231 calories, 8 g total fat, 0 mg cholesterol, 324 mg sodium, 22 g carbohydrate, 2.5 g dietary fiber, 3.5 g protein.*

*Source: USA Dry Pea and Lentil Council, Moscow, Idaho.*

## CHICKEN AND WHITE BEAN SALAD

8 ounces skinless, boneless chicken breast
38-ounce can white beans
1 finely chopped red pepper
2 cloves garlic

Dressing:

1 tablespoon olive oil
1 teaspoon lemon juice
¼ cup balsamic vinegar
½ teaspoon oregano

*Steam, boil, or microwave the chicken until cooked. Shred and place in a large bowl; add beans, red pepper, and garlic, and stir. Combine remaining ingredients together and pour over the chicken and beans and mix thoroughly. Best served chilled. Makes 6 servings.*

Nutrients:

*238 calories, 6 g total fat, 31 g carbohydrate, 11 g dietary fiber, 17 g protein, 57 mg calcium, 3 mg iron.*

Source: University of Utah Nutrition Clinic.

---

## TUNA PASTA SALAD*

¾ cup elbow macaroni, uncooked

6.5-ounce can tuna, water-packed, drained

½ cup celery, thinly sliced

1 cup seedless red grapes, halved

3 tablespoons salad dressing, mayonnaise-type, reduced-calorie

*Cook macaroni according to package directions, omitting salt. Drain. Toss macaroni, tuna, celery, and grapes together. Mix in salad dressing. Serve warm or chill until served. Makes 4 1-cup servings.*

Nutrients:

*195 calories, 2 g fat, trace saturated fatty acids, 13 mg cholesterol, 170 mg sodium.*

Source: United States Department of Agriculture.

# Soups

## BROCCOLI SOUP

1½ cups broccoli, chopped*

¼ cup celery, diced

¼ cup onion, chopped

1 cup chicken broth, unsalted

2 cups skim milk

2 tablespoons cornstarch

¼ teaspoon salt

Dash pepper

Dash ground thyme

¼ cup Swiss cheese, shredded

*Place vegetables and broth in a saucepan. Bring to boiling, reduce heat, cover, and cook until vegetables are tender—about 8 minutes.*

*Mix milk, cornstarch, salt, pepper, and thyme; add to cooked vegetables. Cook, stirring constantly, until soup is slightly thickened and mixture just begins to boil. Remove from heat. Add cheese and stir until melted. Makes 4 1-cup servings.*

*\*Note: A 10-ounce package of frozen, chopped broccoli can be used in place of fresh broccoli. The soup will have about 120 calories and 260 mg of sodium per serving using frozen rather than fresh broccoli.*

*Nutrients:*

*110 calories, 3 g fat, 2 g saturated fatty acids, 9 mg cholesterol, 250 mg sodium.*

*Source: United States Department of Agriculture.*

---

## FISH STEW*

 1 tablespoon olive oil
 1 onion, chopped
 1 sweet green pepper, chopped
 2 cloves garlic, chopped
 1 teaspoon basil
 28-ounce can whole tomatoes (low salt)
 1 can tomato sauce (low salt)
 1 pound cod or other white fish

*Heat oil; add onion and green pepper, cook until soft; add garlic and basil, cook 1 minute. Add tomatoes and sauce; bring to a boil, cut up tomatoes. Simmer 15 minutes. Cut fish into chunks and add to above; simmer until fish is cooked. Serve with rice. Makes 4 to 6 servings.*

---

## WHITE BEAN SOUP*

 ½ pound dry navy beans, rinsed, or canned white beans, rinsed
 2 celery stalks, cut up
 1 carrot, sliced
 1 onion
 1 clove garlic
 1 tablespoon olive oil
 1 large can low-sodium chicken broth
 1 10-ounce package frozen chopped spinach
 ½ cup elbow macaroni or other small pasta

*Bring dry beans to boil in pan of water; boil 5 minutes. Remove from heat. Cover and let stand 1 hour. Drain. Stir fry celery, carrots, onion, and garlic in oil about 5 minutes. Add beans and chicken broth and bring to a boil; cover and simmer until beans are tender—about 1 hour. Add spinach; boil, then simmer until spinach is heated. Add cooked pasta.*

## SPLIT PEA SOUP WITH GREEN HERBS

1 pound USA split peas, rinsed
2 quarts chicken stock or broth
1 large leek, chopped
1 tablespoon lemon juice
1 tablespoon sugar
⅛ teaspoon marjoram
1 pinch nutmeg
⅛ teaspoon thyme
5 ounces spinach, washed and chopped, or frozen
3 tablespoons parsley, chopped
Salt and pepper to taste

*Combine split peas, chicken stock, leek, lemon juice, sugar, and spices. Cook slowly until peas are soft (45 to 60 minutes). Whisk or blend peas until pureed. Ten minutes before serving add spinach and parsley. Adjust consistency; season to taste with salt and pepper. Serves 8 to 10.*

*Nutrients:*

*235 calories, 3 g fat, 2 mg cholesterol, 1,278 mg sodium, 33 g carbohydrate, 3 g dietary fiber, 21 g protein.*

*Source: USA Dry Pea and Lentil Council, Moscow, Idaho.*

## LENTIL AND BARLEY SOUP

1 cup onion, chopped
1 cup celery, chopped
1 clove garlic, minced
¼ cup vegetable oil
6 cups water
28-ounce can tomatoes or 4 cups fresh tomatoes, diced
¾ cup USA lentils, rinsed
¾ cup pearl barley
6 vegetarian bouillon cubes

½ teaspoon dried rosemary, crushed
½ teaspoon dried oregano, crushed
¼ teaspoon pepper
2 cups carrots, thinly sliced
1 cup shredded Swiss cheese, optional

*In a large, heavy soup pot, cook the onions, celery, and garlic in hot oil until tender. Add the water, tomatoes, lentils, barley, bouillon cubes, rosemary, oregano, pepper, and carrots. Cook for 40 minutes, or until the barley, lentils, and carrots are tender. Top with Swiss cheese, if desired. Serves 10.*

*Nutrients:*

*170 calories, 6 g fat, 0 mg cholesterol, 683 mg sodium, 26 g carbohydrate, 6 g dietary fiber, 5 g protein.*

*Source: USA Dry Pea and Lentil Council, Moscow, Idaho.*

## VEGETARIAN SPLIT PEA SOUP—LOW SODIUM

2 cups USA split peas, washed
1 bay leaf
2 quarts water
¼ cup snipped fresh parsley
1 cup celery, sliced
½ teaspoon crushed oregano
½ cup onion, diced
¼ teaspoon crushed basil
1 cup carrots, chopped
1 teaspoon dried Italian seasoning
1 cup potato, diced
½ teaspoon salt
1 clove garlic, minced
Pinch cayenne

*Combine all ingredients in a Dutch oven. Bring to a boil. Reduce heat, cover, and simmer 1 hour or until split peas are cooked through. Remove bay leaf before serving. Makes 10 1-cup servings.*

*Nutrients:*

*118 calories, less than 1 g fat, 139 mg sodium, 22 g carbohydrate, 5 g dietary fiber, 8 g protein.*

*Source: USA Dry Pea and Lentil Council, Moscow, Idaho.*

## SPICY SOUTHWESTERN CHOWDER

2 slices uncooked bacon, chopped
1 medium onion, chopped
1 cup shredded carrots (about 2 medium)
1 to 2 jalapeño peppers, seeded and minced
2 cloves garlic, minced
1½ teaspoons chili powder
½ teaspoon ground cumin
3 cups low-fat milk
2 cups reduced-sodium chicken broth
3 cups cooked brown rice
16-ounce package frozen corn or 17-ounce can corn, drained
6 large sourdough round rolls, hollowed out leaving ½-inch walls
Green onions for garnish

*Cook bacon in Dutch oven over medium-high heat 5 to 7 minutes, stirring until bacon is crisp. Drain all but 1 tablespoon fat. Add onion, carrots, jalapeños, garlic, chili powder, and cumin. Cook 3 to 5 minutes, stirring constantly until onion is tender. Reduce heat to medium. Add milk, broth, rice, and corn. Cook, stirring, 10 to 12 minutes until mixture boils. Cook 1 minute more; remove from heat. Ladle into bread rounds. Garnish with green onions. Makes 6 servings.*

*Nutrients:*

*590 calories, 7 g fat, 15 mg cholesterol, 780 mg sodium, 110 g carbohydrate, 5 g dietary fiber, 20 g protein.*

*Source: USA Rice Council, Houston, Texas.*

---

## MINESTRONE SOUP*

½ cup uncooked regular or whole-wheat macaroni
16-ounce package frozen mixed vegetables
2 cups vegetable broth
15.5-ounce can kidney beans
16-ounce can tomatoes
2 tablespoons chopped parsley

*Cook macaroni in boiling water for 10 minutes; drain. Chop vegetables; cook in vegetable broth for 15 minutes. Add beans, tomatoes, and macaroni. Add seasonings to taste. Makes 8 servings.*

*Nutrients:*

*142 calories, 1.5 g fat, 26 g carbohydrate, 6 g fiber, 7 g protein, 38 mg calcium, 1.5 mg iron.*
*Source: University of Utah Nutrition Clinic.*

---

## VEGETABLE SOUP*

8-ounce can low-salt tomato sauce
1 cup water
Salt to taste
2 potatoes, sliced
1 zucchini, sliced
3 carrots, sliced
1 teaspoon basil

*In saucepan, stir together tomato sauce, water, and salt. Add sliced vegetables and basil and bring to boil. Cook on low heat, covered, until vegetables are tender.*

---

## MEATLESS LENTIL CHILI

2½ cups (1 pound) USA lentils, rinsed
5 cups water
1-ounce packet dry onion soup mix
16-ounce can tomatoes or tomato sauce
1½ teaspoons chili powder
½ teaspoon cumin

*In a large saucepan, bring lentils and water to a boil. Add dry onion soup mix and simmer for 30 minutes. Add the rest of the ingredients and simmer 30 minutes longer. Serve over spaghetti, rice, or corn chips. Garnish with cheese. Chili can also be used on pizzas, in tacos, or as a dip. Serves 6 to 8.*

*Nutrients:*

*210 calories, trace of fat, 333 mg cholesterol, 1,129 mg sodium, 40 g carbohydrate, 9 g dietary fiber, 14 g protein.*

*Source: USA Dry Pea and Lentil Council, Moscow, Idaho.*

---

## NORTHWEST LENTIL CHILI

32-ounce can (4 cups) tomato juice
½ cup diced onion
2 cups diced, raw potato

2 tablespoon chili powder
15-ounce can garbanzo beans
2 teaspoons beef bouillon granules
1 cup USA lentils, washed
1 teaspoon crushed basil
1 cup diced carrots
2 cloves garlic, minced

*Combine all ingredients in a Dutch oven and bring to a boil. Reduce heat and simmer, covered, about 30 minutes or until lentils are tender. Makes 10 1-cup servings.*

*Nutrients:*

*152 calories, 1 g fat, 544 mg sodium, 29 g carbohydrate, 6 g dietary fiber, 9 g protein.*

*Source: USA Dry Pea and Lentil Council, Moscow, Idaho.*

# Rice

## RICE OLÉ

1 cup chopped onions
1 cup chopped green peppers
½ cup celery, finely chopped
1 tablespoon butter or margarine
1 teaspoon chili powder
1 teaspoon garlic salt
14.5-ounce can peeled whole tomatoes, chopped
3 cups cooked rice

*Combine onions, peppers, celery, and butter in 2½-quart microwave-proof baking dish. Cover and cook on high 6 minutes. Add seasonings, tomatoes, and rice; stir. Cover and cook on high 4 minutes. Let stand 5 minutes. Makes 6 servings.*

*Nutrients:*

*128 calories, 2 g fat, 5 mg cholesterol, 489 mg sodium, 24 g carbohydrate, 3 g protein.*

*Source: USA Rice Council, Houston, Texas.*

## SPANISH RICE

1½ cups uncooked brown rice
2½ cups water
2½ teaspoons seasoning salt

1 cup onion, chopped

½ cup green peppers

2 tablespoons corn oil

½ teaspoon garlic powder

½ cup tomatoes, diced, canned in puree

2 tablespoons tomato paste

½ teaspoon cumin

1 teaspoon salt

*Cook rice in water with seasoning salt until tender (approximately 50 minutes). Sauté onions and green pepper in oil. Add garlic powder. Add remaining ingredients and cook for 5 minutes, stirring frequently. Add cooked rice. Mix well and simmer 3 to 4 minutes, stirring occasionally.*

Source: Loma Linda University.

# Poultry

## CHICKEN DIJON*

¼ cup Dijon-style mustard

¼ cup low-fat or fat-free mayonnaise

2 chicken breasts (skinned, halved)

1 cup cornflake crumbs

⅓ cup Parmesan cheese

*Blend mayonnaise and mustard and coat chicken; roll in crumbs. Cover with cheese and bake at 325° F. for 1 hour. Serves 2.*

## CURRY CHICKEN*

1 pound boneless, skinless chicken breasts or thighs, chunked

1 tablespoon olive oil

1 onion, chopped

4 cloves garlic, sliced thin

2 teaspoons curry powder (more if you like it a little spicier)

¼ teaspoon ground ginger

⅛ teaspoon salt

½ cup chopped tomatoes

⅓ cup water

*Sauté chicken in oil until browned all over. Put chicken in bowl; pat up excess oil with paper towels, and keep chicken warm. Lower heat and add onion and garlic to pan. Cook, stirring frequently, until lightly browned and soft. Stir in curry powder, ginger, and salt; cook 1 minute. Stir in tomatoes and water; cook 1 minute more.  Add chicken; bring to boiling. Lower heat; cover and simmer until chicken is cooked and no pink remains. Serve over rice, with chopped nuts, parsley, raisins, or low-fat yogurt.*

## ITALIAN CHICKEN*

4 chicken breast halves, skinned
½ teaspoon oregano leaves
¼ teaspoon basil leaves
½ cup onion, chopped
⅛ teaspoon garlic powder
½ medium green pepper, chopped
⅛ teaspoon salt
2 8-ounce cans no-salt-added tomato sauce

*Brown chicken in hot frying pan. Mix the rest of the ingredients together and pour the mixture over chicken. Heat the mixture until it boils, then reduce the heat, cover, and cook over low heat until chicken is tender, about 45 minutes. Makes 4 servings of ½ breast and ½ cup sauce each.*

*Nutrients:*

*190 calories, 2 g fat, 70 mg cholesterol, 180 mg sodium.*

*Source: United States Department of Agriculture.*

## TURKEY CASSEROLE*

6-ounce package wild rice or wild rice and white rice mix
½ cup chopped onion
½ cup chopped celery
1–2 tablespoons olive oil
1 can whole cranberries
3 tablespoons white grape juice
1 teaspoon white wine vinegar
2 cups cooked, chopped turkey

*Prepare rice according to package directions. Cook onion and celery in oil until tender. Stir in cranberries, grape juice, and vinegar. Stir in turkey and rice. Put in baking dish. Bake covered at 350° F. for 35 to 45 minutes. Stir.*

# Seafood

## BROILED SESAME FISH

For a quick, low-fat main dish, try this fish recipe. It takes about 15 minutes to prepare and contains very little fat.

I pound cod fillets, fresh or frozen
I teaspoon margarine, melted
I tablespoon lemon juice
I teaspoon dried tarragon leaves
⅛ teaspoon salt
Dash pepper
I tablespoon sesame seed
I tablespoon parsley, chopped

*Thaw frozen fish in refrigerator overnight or defrost briefly in a microwave oven. Cut fish into four portions. Place fish on a broiler pan lined with aluminum foil. Brush margarine over fish. Mix lemon juice, tarragon leaves, salt, and pepper. Pour over fish. Sprinkle sesame seeds evenly over fish. Broil until fish flakes easily when tested with a fork— about 12 minutes. Garnish each serving with parsley. Makes 4 2.5-ounce servings.*

Nutrients:

110 calories, 3 g fat, trace saturated fatty acids, 46 mg cholesterol, 155 mg sodium.

Source: United States Department of Agriculture.

---

## FISH PARMESAN*

1½ pounds filleted fish
garlic salt
pepper
½ teaspoon oregano
8-ounce jar marinara sauce
grated mozzarella cheese
2 tablespoons Parmesan cheese

*Season fish with garlic salt, pepper, and oregano. Put fish in baking dish. Pour marinara sauce over it. Sprinkle with cheeses and bake at 425° F. for 15 minutes. Serves 4.*

## SHRIMP PITA

¾ cup olive oil
½ cup red wine vinegar
2 medium onions, chopped, divided
2 cloves garlic, minced, divided
2 teaspoons Italian seasoning, divided
1 pound medium shrimp, peeled, each cut in half and deveined
2 medium-sized red or green bell peppers, julienned
4 cups fresh spinach leaves, stems removed and torn
3 cups cooked brown rice
1 teaspoon salt
½ teaspoon ground black pepper
3 6-inch pita breads

*Combine oil, vinegar, ½ cup chopped onion, 1 clove garlic, and 1 teaspoon Italian seasoning in large bowl. Add shrimp; stir until well coated. Cover and refrigerate 4 hours or overnight. Thoroughly drain shrimp; discard marinade. Heat large skillet over medium-high heat until hot. Add shrimp, remaining onion, bell peppers, spinach, and remaining 1 clove garlic; sauté 3 to 5 minutes or until shrimp is no longer pink and spinach is wilted. Add rice, remaining teaspoon Italian seasoning, salt, and pepper. Cook and stir 2 to 3 minutes or until flavors are well blended. To serve, fill each pita with ½- to ¾-cup rice. Makes 6 servings.*

*Nutrients:*

*296 calories, 6 g fat, 61 mg cholesterol, 677 mg sodium, 47 g carbohydrate, 6 g dietary fiber, 14 g protein.*

*Source: USA Rice Council, Houston, Texas.*

# Meatless Entrées

## VEGETABLE QUESADILLAS*

1 red pepper, raw
1 yellow pepper, raw
1 carrot, raw

4 scallions
2 cups tomatoes, chopped
4 tablespoons hot picante salsa
I cup plain nonfat yogurt
4 corn tortillas
8 ounces part-skim mozzarella cheese
8 pieces iceberg lettuce

*Chop the vegetables and mix together. Combine salsa and yogurt, set aside. Arrange vegetables on the corn tortillas, top with cheese, and fold in half. Microwave on high for about 40 seconds. Top with lettuce and salsa–yogurt mixture. Makes 4 servings.*

*Nutrients:*

*313 calories, 30% DV fat, 33 mg cholesterol, 524 mg sodium, 39% DV carbohydrate, 31% DV protein, 618 mg calcium, 2 mg iron.*

*Source: University of Utah Nutrition Clinic.*

---

## BROWN RICE–BLACK BEAN BURRITO

I tablespoon vegetable oil
I medium onion, chopped
2 cloves garlic, minced
1½ teaspoons chili powder
½ teaspoon cumin
3 cups cooked brown rice
15- to 16-ounce can black beans, drained and rinsed
11-ounce can corn, drained
6 (8-inch) flour tortillas
¾ cup (6 ounces) shredded reduced-fat cheddar cheese
2 green onions, thinly sliced
¼ cup plain low-fat yogurt
¼ cup prepared salsa

*Heat oil in large skillet over medium-high heat until hot. Add onion, garlic, chili powder, and cumin. Sauté 3 to 5 minutes or until onion is tender. Add rice, beans, and corn; cook, stirring 2 to 3 minutes until mixture is thoroughly heated. Remove from heat. Spoon ½ cup rice mixture down center of each tortilla. Top each with 2 tablespoons cheese, I tablespoon green onion, and I tablespoon yogurt; roll up, top with I tablespoon salsa. Makes 6 servings.*

*Nutrients:*

*456 calories, 9 g fat, 10 mg cholesterol, 591 mg sodium, 73 g carbohydrate, 6 g dietary fiber, 23 g protein.*

*Source: USA Rice Council, Houston, Texas.*

---

## BAGEL PIZZA*

1 bagel

On each half place:

1 tablespoon pre-made pizza sauce
1½ ounces mozzarella cheese
sliced tomatoes
mushrooms
red onions
*Bake at 400° F. for 4 to 5 minutes.*

---

# Beef

## BEEF AND VEGETABLE STIR FRY

¾ pound (12 ounces) beef round steak, boneless
1 teaspoon vegetable oil
½ cup carrots, sliced
¼ cup celery, sliced
½ cup onion, sliced
⅛ teaspoon garlic powder
Dash pepper
1 tablespoon soy sauce
2 cups zucchini squash, cut in thin strips
1 tablespoon cornstarch
¼ cup water

*Trim all fat from steak. Slice steak across the grain into thin strips about ⅛-inch wide and 3 inches long. (Partially frozen meat is easier to slice.) Heat oil in frying pan. Add beef strips and stir fry over high heat, turning pieces constantly, until beef is no longer red—about 3 to 5 minutes. Reduce heat. Add carrots, celery, onion, and seasonings. Cover and cook until carrots are slightly tender—3 to 4 minutes. Add squash; cook until vegetables are tender-crisp—3 to 4 minutes. Mix cornstarch* and water until smooth; add slowly to beef mixture, stirring constantly. Cook until thickened and vegetables are coated with a thin glaze. Makes 4 ¾-cup servings.  You may substitute 12 ounces of raw chicken for the beef if desired.

Nutrients:

145 calories, 4 g fat, 1 g saturated fatty acids, 44 mg cholesterol, 300 mg sodium.

With chicken, each serving provides: 140 calories, 2 g fat, trace saturated fatty acids, 51 mg cholesterol, 320 mg sodium.

Source: United States Department of Agriculture.

## SPICY STEAK STRIPS

¾ pound (12 ounces) beef round steak, boneless
½ cup celery, sliced
½ cup onion, chopped
1 tablespoon flour
1 tablespoon Worcestershire sauce
½ teaspoon ginger root, minced
¼ teaspoon salt
16-ounce can tomatoes
⅛ teaspoon ground cloves
½ cup water
⅛ teaspoon red pepper flakes
2 tablespoons parsley, chopped
1 bay leaf

Trim all fat from steak. Slice across the grain diagonally into thin strips. (Partially frozen meat is easier to slice.) Heat nonstick frying pan. Cook steak, celery, and onion until steak is browned. Drain off fat.  Stir flour into beef mixture.  Add remaining ingredients. Bring to a boil; reduce heat, cover, and cook over low heat for 40 minutes or until meat is tender.  Remove bay leaf. Serve over noodles or rice. Makes 4 ½-cup servings.

Nutrients (not including noodles or rice):

140 calories, 3 g fat, 1 g saturated fatty acids, 43 mg cholesterol, 245 mg sodium.

Source: United States Department of Agriculture.

# Sauces and Dips

## HOMEMADE PASTA SAUCE*

3 cloves garlic, crushed
Fresh or canned mushrooms
1 small zucchini or yellow squash, sliced
2 tablespoons olive oil
1 to 2 28-ounce cans crushed tomatoes or fresh skinned tomatoes
3 tablespoons chopped fresh basil

*Sauté garlic, mushrooms, and zucchini in oil. Add tomatoes; cook uncovered until slightly thickened. Stir in basil.*

---

## CHILI BEAN DIP

15-ounce can kidney beans
3 tablespoons drained bean liquid
1 tablespoon vinegar
⅛ teaspoon ground cumin
1 teaspoon chili powder
2 teaspoons onion, grated
2 teaspoons parsley, chopped

*Drain kidney beans; save liquid. Place drained beans, bean liquid, vinegar, and seasonings in blender. Blend until smooth. Remove mixture from blender. Stir in onion and parsley. Chill thoroughly. Serve with crisp vegetable sticks. Makes about 1⅓ cups.*

*Nutrients (per tablespoon):*

*15 calories, trace fat, trace saturated fatty acids, 0 mg cholesterol, 55 mg sodium.*

*Source: United States Department of Agriculture.*

---

## HOT 'N' SPICY SEASONING

¼ cup paprika
1 teaspoon black pepper
2 tablespoons oregano
½ teaspoon red pepper
2 teaspoons chili powder
½ teaspoon dry mustard
1 teaspoon garlic powder

*Mix all of the above in a bowl. Store in an airtight container.*

*This seasoning tastes good on meat, poultry, or fish. Instead of salt, sprinkle some on the food, and then cook it as you usually do. Or, mix some with plain breadcrumbs and then coat the meat with the crumbs. If you like it very spicy, use more.*

*Source: National Institute of Health.*

---

## CHEESE SAUCE FOR BROCCOLI AND CAULIFLOWER

4 tablespoons margarine or butter

4 tablespoons flour

2 cups skim milk

1 cup low-fat or non-fat grated cheese—any yellow cheese

*Steam broccoli and cauliflower until tender.*

*Melt margarine or butter in frying pan. Add flour and stir. Add milk; stir on low heat until thickened. Add grated cheese; stir until melted.*

*Put cauliflower and broccoli in baking dish; pour cheese sauce on top and bake at 300° F. for 30 minutes.*

# Cereals and Breads

## GRANOLA*

6 cups rolled oats

1 cup roasted sunflower seeds

1 cup wheat germ

1 cup roasted almonds, chopped

1 cup unprocessed bran

1½ cups raisins

*Mix above ingredients together and store in an airtight container. If desired, cereal can be toasted on a greased cookie sheet for 20 minutes in a 300° F. oven. Makes approximately 20 ½-cup servings.*

*Nutrients:*

*246 calories, 34% DV fat, 0 mg cholesterol, 55 mg sodium, 51% DV carbohydrate, 15% DV protein, 45 mg calcium, 3 mg iron.*

*Source: University of Utah Nutrition Clinic.*

## BLENDER PANCAKES

1 cup wheat, uncooked
1½ cups milk*
1 teaspoon salt
1 tablespoon baking powder
1 egg
2 tablespoons oil
3 tablespoons sugar

*Combine wheat and 1 cup of milk in blender. Blend on high for 1 minute. Add remaining ingredients and blend until smooth. Cook on hot griddle. Serve with favorite topping. Makes 6 to 8 servings.*

*\*Dry milk may be substituted. Add 4 tablespoons non-instant powdered milk or ½ cup instant milk powder to wheat. Then use the same amount of water as called for with fresh milk.*

Nutrients:

175 calories, 6 g fat, 33 mg cholesterol, 453 mg sodium, 24 g carbohydrate, 1 g dietary fiber, 6 g protein.

Source: Utah State University Extension, Salt Lake County.

## SWEET GINGERCRISP

⅓ cup maple syrup
¼ cup lemon juice
3 tablespoons water
1 teaspoon vanilla extract
4 cups sliced unpeeled apples
3 cups cooked brown rice
vegetable cooking spray
2 tablespoons all-purpose flour
2 tablespoons brown sugar, packed
1 teaspoon allspice
2 tablespoons butter or margarine
¾ cup coarsely crushed gingersnap cookies (about 10)
1 cup nonfat vanilla yogurt, divided

*Combine maple syrup, lemon juice, water, and vanilla in large bowl. Stir in apples and rice. Spoon into casserole dish coated with cooking spray. Combine flour, brown sugar, and allspice in small bowl; cut in butter until crumbly. Stir in gingersnaps and sprinkle over apples and rice.*

*Bake covered in 400° F. oven for 35 minutes. Remove cover, bake 10 minutes more or until top is golden brown and apples are tender. Serve warm, topping each serving with 1 tablespoon yogurt. Makes 8 servings.*

Nutrients:

*268 calories, 5 g fat, 12 mg cholesterol, 210 mg sodium, 52 g carbohydrate, 2 g dietary fiber, 4 g protein.*

*Source: USA Rice Council, Houston, Texas.*

---

## APPLE CRISP

4 cups tart apples, pared, sliced
¼ cup water
1 tablespoon lemon juice
¼ cup brown sugar, packed
¼ cup whole-wheat flour
¼ cup old-fashioned rolled oats
½ teaspoon ground cinnamon
¼ teaspoon ground nutmeg
3 tablespoons margarine

*Place apples in 8" x 8" x 2" baking pan. Mix water and lemon juice; pour over apples. Mix sugar, flour, oats, and spices. Add margarine to dry mixture; mix until crumbly. Sprinkle crumbly mixture evenly over apples. Bake at 350° F. until apples are tender and topping is lightly browned, about 40 minutes. Makes 4 ½-cup servings.*

Nutrients:

*235 calories, 9 g fat, 2 g saturated fatty acids, 0 mg cholesterol, 105 mg sodium.*

*Source: United States Department of Agriculture.*

---

## FRUIT BRAN MUFFINS*

2½ cups bran cereal
1½ cups skim milk
4 egg whites
1 tablespoon vanilla
2 cups flour
½ cup brown sugar
1½ teaspoons cinnamon
2 tablespoons baking powder
¾ teaspoon baking soda
2 cups fresh or frozen fruit or dried cranberries or cherries

Preheat oven to 325° F. Combine cereal, milk, egg whites, and vanilla. Stir together flour, brown sugar, cinnamon, baking powder, and baking soda. Combine dry and wet mixtures. Fold in fruit. Spoon into paper-lined muffin tins. Bake for 30 minutes.

Nutrients:

141 calories, 4% DV fat, 82% DV carbohydrates, 14% DV protein.

Source: University of Utah Nutrition Clinic.

## PUMPKIN CUPCAKES

   1½ cups whole-wheat flour
   1 cup all-purpose flour
   ¾ cup sugar
   2 tablespoons baking powder
   2 teaspoons ground cinnamon
   ½ teaspoon ground nutmeg
   ¼ teaspoon salt
   3 eggs, slightly beaten
   1 cup skim milk
   ½ cup vegetable oil
   1 cup canned pumpkin
   ¾ cup raisins, chopped
   1 tablespoon vanilla

Preheat oven to 350° F. Place 24 paper baking cups in muffin tins. Mix dry ingredients thoroughly. Mix remaining ingredients; add to dry ingredients. Stir until dry ingredients are barely moistened. Fill paper cups two-thirds full. Bake about 20 minutes or until toothpick inserted in center comes out clean. Remove from muffin tins and cool on rack. Freeze cupcakes that will not be eaten in the next few days. Makes 24 cupcakes.

Nutrients (per cupcake):

140 calories, 5 g fat, 1 g saturated fatty acids, 27 mg cholesterol, 130 mg sodium.

Source: United States Department of Agriculture.

## OATMEAL APPLESAUCE COOKIES

   1 cup all-purpose flour
   1 teaspoon baking powder
   1 teaspoon ground allspice

¼ teaspoon salt
½ cup margarine
½ cup sugar
2 egg whites
2 cups rolled oats, quick-cooking
1 cup unsweetened applesauce
½ cup raisins, chopped

*Preheat oven to 375° F. Grease baking sheet. Mix flour, baking powder, allspice, and salt. Beat margarine and sugar until creamy. Add egg whites; beat well. Add dry ingredients. Stir in oats, applesauce, and raisins. Mix well. Drop by level tablespoonfuls onto baking sheet. Bake 11 minutes or until edges are lightly browned. Cool on rack. Makes about 5 dozen cookies.*

*Nutrients (per cookie):*

*45 calories, 2 g fat, trace saturated fatty acids, 0 mg cholesterol, 35 mg sodium.*

*Source: United States Department of Agriculture.*

## ZUCCHINI BREAD

1 cup whole-wheat flour
1 cup all-purpose flour
1½ teaspoons baking powder
1 teaspoon ground cinnamon
¼ teaspoon baking soda
¼ teaspoon salt
3 egg whites
½ cup sugar
⅓ cup vegetable oil
1½ teaspoons vanilla
2 cups zucchini squash, coarsely shredded, lightly packed

*Preheat oven to 350° F. Grease 9" x 5" x 3" loaf pan. Mix dry ingredients, except sugar. Beat egg whites until frothy. Add sugar, oil, and vanilla. Continue beating for 3 minutes. Stir in zucchini; mix lightly. Add dry ingredients. Mix just until dry ingredients are moistened. Pour into loaf pan. Bake 40 minutes or until toothpick inserted in center comes out clean. Cool on rack. Remove from pan after 10 minutes. To serve, cut into 18 slices about ½-inch thick. Makes 1 loaf.*

*Nutrients (per slice):*

*110 calories, 4 g fat, 1 g saturated fatty acids, 0 mg cholesterol, 90 mg sodium.*

*Source: United States Department of Agriculture.*

---

## BRAN APPLE BARS

Apples and bran cereal add dietary fiber. Using egg whites in place of a whole egg keeps cholesterol to a trace.

    1 cup whole-bran cereal*
    ½ cup skim milk
    1 cup flour
    1 teaspoon baking powder
    ½ teaspoon ground cinnamon
    ¼ teaspoon ground nutmeg
    ⅓ cup margarine
    ½ cup brown sugar, packed
    2 egg whites
    1 cup apple, pared, chopped

*Preheat oven to 350° F. Grease 9" x 9" baking pan. Soak bran in milk until milk is absorbed. Mix dry ingredients thoroughly. Beat margarine and sugar until creamy. Add egg whites; beat well. Stir in apples and bran mixture. Add dry ingredients; mix well. Pour into pan. Bake 30 minutes or until a toothpick inserted in center comes out clean. Cool on rack. Cut into 16 bars.*

*\* Note: Check the nutrition label of cereals for sodium content. Some whole-bran cereals contain almost twice as much sodium as others.*

*Nutrients (per bar):*

*110 calories, 4 g fat, 1 g saturated fatty acids, trace cholesterol, 110 mg sodium.*

*Source: United States Department of Agriculture.*

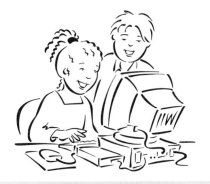

# WEB SITES

**www.americanhiking.org** Web site of the American Hiking Society. Provides information on local trails, including length and difficulty.

**www.nationaleatingdisorders.org** Web site for eating disorders.

**www.ext.usu.edu** Web site of Utah State University Extension. Provides nutritional information, recipes.

**www.fitness.gov** President's Council on Physical Fitness and Sports Web site. Provides information on fitness for kids and adults.

**www.health.org/gpower** Web site of the U.S. Department of Health and Human Services to encourage girls ages 9 to 13 to adopt healthier lifestyles.

**www.caprojectlean.org** Web site of the California Public Health Institute's "Project Lean."

**www.niddk.nih.gov/health/nutrit** The National Institutes of Health Weight Control Information Network.

**www.eatright.org** Web site of the American Dietetic Association.

**www.aap.org/family** Web site of the American Academy of Pediatrics.

**www.nal.usda.gov/fnic** U.S. Department of Agriculture—Food and Nutrition Information Center.

**www.ific.org** Web site of the International Food Information Council. Provides information on child and adult nutrition and food additives, pesticides, and bioengineering.

185

**www.americanheart.org** Web site of the American Heart Association.

**www.usda.gov/fcs/team.htm** Web site for Team Nutrition. Provides nutrition resources for teachers, students, parents, and school lunch providers.

**www.dole5aday.com** Dole Web site, provides a kid's cookbook.

**www.5aday.gov** Web site for the National Cancer Institute.

**www.5aday.com** Web site of Produce for Better Health.

**www.hearthighway.org** Fun activities and lesson plans for teachers and students, from the Utah Department of Health, Cardiovascular Program.

**www.cdc.gov** Web site for Centers for Disease Control and Prevention.

**www.fourhcouncil.edu** Web site for the Four H Club.

**www.nationaldairycouncil.org** Web site of the National Dairy Council.

**www.nhlbi.nih.gov** Web site of the National Heart, Lung, Blood Institute. Provides general information on cardiovascular disease.

**www.mayohealth.org** The Mayo Clinic Health Oasis Web site. Provides diet and nutrition information and a virtual cookbook.

**www.navigator.tufts.edu** Web site of Tufts University. Provides links to nutrition-related web sites.

**www.pueblo.gsa.gov** Web site of the Consumer Information Center. Go to the Food and Nutrition section and the Diet and Exercise part of the Health section.

**www.cfsan.fda.gov/list.html** Web site of the U.S. Food and Drug Administration. Provides information on fat and fiber in the Nutrition and Dietary Guidelines section. The Losing Weight and Maintaining a Healthy Weight link provides information on weight loss scams.

**www.diabetes.org** Web site of the American Diabetes Association.

**www.vrg.org** Web site of the Vegetarian Resource Group. Provides information on healthy diets without meat.

**www.eatethnic.com** Web site for Eat Ethnic. Provides information on cultural foods.

**www.foodsafety.org** Web site for the National Food Safety Database.

Web sites that charge a fee for customized diets and exercise plans:

www.MealsForYou.com

www.cyberdiet.com

www.eDiets.com

www.Nutricise.com

www.DietWatch.com

www.Weightwatchers.com

www.shapeup.org

YOU MET YOUR WEEKLY GOAL.
WAY TO GO!

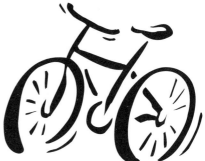

NAME _____

DATE _____

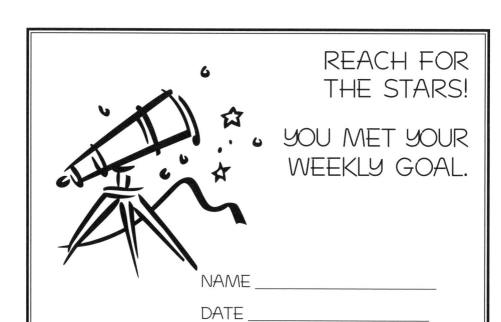

REACH FOR
THE STARS!

YOU MET YOUR
WEEKLY GOAL.

NAME _____

DATE _____

YOU MET YOUR
WEEKLY GOAL.

KEEP IT UP!

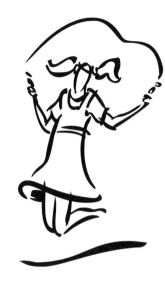

NAME _____

DATE _____

YOU MET YOUR WEEKLY GOAL.
CLAIM YOUR MEDAL OF HONOR!

NAME _____

DATE _____

YOU MET YOUR WEEKLY GOAL.
WAY TO GO!

NAME _____

DATE _____

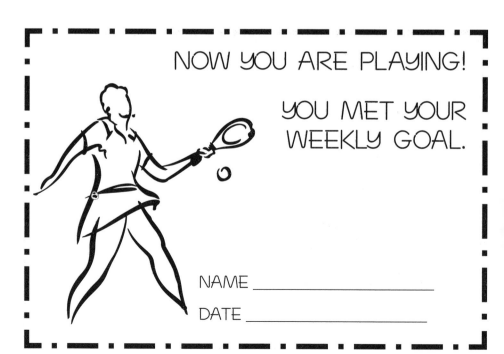

NOW YOU ARE PLAYING!

YOU MET YOUR
WEEKLY GOAL.

NAME _____

DATE _____

# CERTIFICATE OF COMPLETION

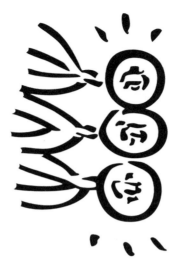

_____

HAS SUCCESSFULLY COMPLETED

THE HEALTHY FAMILY PROGRAM

DATE _____

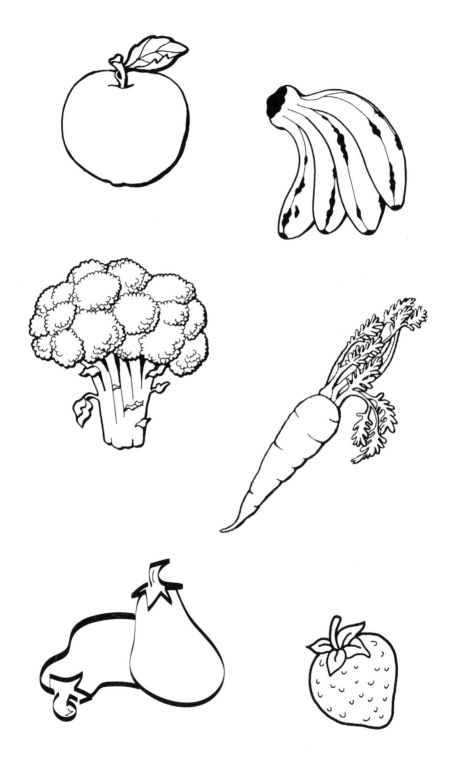

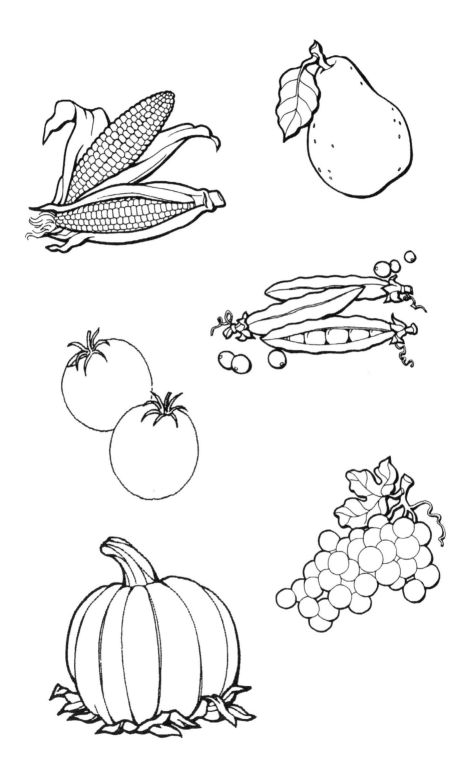

# INDEX